INTRODUCTION

Companion Text Book

This study workbook utilizes the text book - Cloherty and Stark's Manual of Neonatal Care, Eighth Edition by Eric C. Eichenwald, Anne R. Hansen, Camilia R. Martin and Ann R. Stark as the core study text. ISBN 978-1-4963-4361-1, published by Wolters Kluwer, Philadelphia PA, 2017.

How to Use this Workbook and Practice Text

- Choose and read a chapter in the textbook.
- Complete the workbook exercises associated with the chapter you are studying.
- Mark any exercises you can't readily answer.
- Go back to the textbook and find the answer to the exercises you didn't know. (Textbook page references are cited.)
- Complete this process for all the chapters. Once completed, re-review the exercises concentrating on the content that was most challenging.
- After you have reviewed the information and feel confident of your knowledge, complete the practice test at the back of the workbook. (Answers are provided.)

NCC Certification Competencies

To see the test outline and associated competencies for the Neonatal Intensive Care Nursing, Neonatal Nurse Practitioner or Low Risk Neonatal Intensive Care Nursing NCC certification examinations, please refer to the NCC Candidate Guides posted on **NCCwebsite.org**.

Continuing Education (CE)

Purchase and successfully complete the companion continuing education post-test to earn 30 CE hours for licensure and/or NCC maintenance.

Visit the Test Center at CCPRwebsite.org.

If you plan to use CCPR CE for your NCC maintenance, it is recommended that you do not complete this CE post-test until after you have passed your NCC certification exam and completed your NCC continuing competency assessment.

CCPR CE tests are: Provider approved by the California Board of Nursing Provider #15130.

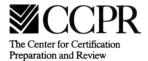

CCPR Neonatal Nursing Study Workbook with Practice Test
ISBN: 978-0-9890938-6-6

©2021 The Center for Certification Preparation and Review
All Rights Reserved. No part of this publication may be reproduced or transmitted by any means, electronic or mechanical, including photocopying, recording or otherwise, without written permission from the publisher. For information, write The Center for Certification Preparation and Review, 676 N. Michigan Ave, Suite 3600, Chicago, IL 60611.

DISCLAIMER

CCPR is an independent not-for-profit organization and is solely responsible for the development of this Study Workbook for Certification Review. Utilization of the Study Workbook to prepare for NCC certification does not imply a guarantee that certification will be achieved.

Every effort is made to insure the information contained in the CCPR Study Workbook for Certification Review is accurate; however, CCPR disclaims any responsibility for any errors or omissions it may contain.

The book and the individual contributions contained in it are protected by copyright by the Publisher *(Except as noted herein)*.

While all reasonable effort has been made to assure both the accuracy and timeliness of the information in this publication, new evidence and research continually impact practice. The authors, editors and publishers do not take responsibility for the accuracy or completeness of any of the information contained herein and it is expected that providers utilize the most current information, policies and guidelines at their practice sites for the care of patients.

This book and the authors, editors, and publishers recognize that this publication contains information on health care that is intended for use as assistance only to the professional practitioner. The actual use of, and interpretation of, this information is solely the responsibility of the practitioner.

Any reference to any procedure, device, drug, or drug dosage (unless otherwise indicated in the text) is based on the generally accepted standards in effect at the time of publication and, if applicable, reflects the then current FDA-approved usages for drugs and devices. Since such standards and usages are subject to change and interpretation based on research and new information, it is the responsibility of any practitioner to check the applicable current standards and FDA usage recommendations prior to use in practice. The editors, authors, and publisher disclaim any responsibility for any adverse effects resulting from the suggested procedures, from any undetected errors, or from the reader's misunderstanding of the text.

ACKNOWLEDGEMENTS

CCPR acknowledges the contributions of the following authors and reviewers:
Nicole L. Barrett, MSN, ARNP, NNP-BC
Erma Cooke, RN, MS, NNP-BC
Angela Craft, NNP-BC
Marilyn Patterson, MSN, RNC-NIC

Developmental Editor: Cyndi Scovel

Printed in the United States of America
676 N. Michigan Ave., Suite 3600 • Chicago, IL 60611 • info@CCPRwebsite.org

TABLE OF CONTENTS

PART 1	PRENATAL ASSESSMENTS AND CONDITIONS	4
PART 2	ASSESSMENT AND TREATMENT IN THE IMMEDIATE POSTNATAL PERIOD	6
PART 3	GENERAL NEWBORN CONDITIONS	14
PART 4	FLUID ELECTROLYTES, NUTRITION, GASTROINTESTINAL & RENAL ISSUES	24
PART 5	RESPIRATORY DISORDERS	46
PART 6	CARDIOVASCULAR DISORDERS	58
PART 7	HEMATOLOGIC DISORDERS	73
PART 8	INFECTIOUS DISEASES	84
PART 9	NEUROLOGIC DISORDERS	90
PART 10	BONE CONDITIONS	99
PART 11	METABOLISM	102
PART 12	ENDOCRINOLOGY	104
PART 13	SURGERY	109
PART 14	DERMATOLOGY	115
PART 15	VASCULAR ANOMALIES	117
PART 16	AUDITORY AND OPTHALMOLOGIC DISORDERS	119
PART 17	COMMON NEONATAL PROCEDURES	122
PART 18	PAIN AND STRESS CONTROL	124
	STUDY WORKBOOK PRACTICE TEST	126

PART 1 - PRENATAL ASSESSMENT AND CONDITIONS

CHAPTER 1
Fetal Assessment and Prenatal Diagnosis

Indicate if the following statements are true (T) or or false (F) regarding prenatal diagnosis tests.

_____ The best time for alpha-fetoprotein screening is between 15-22 weeks gestation.

_____ High alpha-fetoprotein levels are associated with chromosomal abnormalities.

_____ Nuchal lucency screening is useful in diagnosing trisomy 21 risk.

_____ A negative CST is more reassuring than a reactive NST.

_____ The biophysical profile is determined by measurement of five different parameters.

Text Reference, pages 2-10

Match the electronic fetal monitor terms listed below with the following.

A. Bradycardia   _____ Results from cord compression

B. Tachycardia   _____ May result from congenital heart block

C. Early decelerations   _____ Associated with uteroplacental insufficiency

D. Late decelerations   _____ Mirrors uterine contractions in time of onset, duration and termination

E. Variable decelerations   _____ Can occur with maternal fever

Text Reference, pages 11-12

List three associated etiologies of Fetal Growth Restriction (FGR):

1. _____
2. _____
3. _____

Text Reference, page 7

CHAPTER 2
Maternal Diabetes Mellitus

See workbook Chapter 62 Neonatal Effects of Maternal Diabetes, page 105

CHAPTER 3
Preeclampsia and Related Conditions

Name three implications for infants born to mothers with moderate or severe preeclampsia.

1. _____
2. _____
3. _____

Text Reference, pages 31-32

Neonates born to preeclamptic women who received magnesium sulfate in the intrapartum period are at risk for: *(check all that apply)*

- ❏ Abnormalities of calcium homeostasis
- ❏ Hypoglycemia
- ❏ Hyperbilirubinemia
- ❏ Hypotonia
- ❏ Hypomagnesemia
- ❏ Parathyroid abnormalities

Text Reference, pages 31-32

PART 2 – ASSESSMENT AND TREATMENT IN THE IMMEDIATE POSTNATAL PERIOD

CHAPTER 4

Resuscitation in the Delivery Room

What would be the physical presentation of an infant with an Apgar score of 6?

Text Reference, pages 39 & 49

Differentiate primary from secondary apnea.

Text Reference, pages 40-41

When resuscitating a newborn, how is adequacy of ventilation determined?

Text Reference, page 42

What are the guidelines for initiation of chest compressions and depth for compressions?

What is the correct rate and depth for the compressions?

Text Reference Page 43

What is the recommended dose and strength of epinephrine for neonatal resuscitation?

Text Reference, pages 44-45 Table 4.3 & page 46

When should administration of volume expanders be considered?

Text Reference, pages 46-47

Discuss the significance of Apgar scoring.

Text Reference, pages 48-49

Discuss withholding or withdrawing resuscitation.

Text Reference, page 50

PART 2 – ASSESSMENT AND TREATMENT IN THE IMMEDIATE POSTNATAL PERIOD

CHAPTER 5

Nonimmune Hydrops Fetalis

List five etiologies of nonimmune hydrops fetalis:

1. _____
2. _____
3. _____
4. _____
5. _____

Text Reference, page 55

Discuss the delivery room management of Fetal Hydrops.

_____
_____
_____

Text Reference, page 61

CHAPTER 6

Birth Trauma

Identify at least five risk factors for birth trauma:

1. _____
2. _____
3. _____
4. _____
5. _____

Text Reference, page 64-65

Indicate if the following statements about birth trauma are true (**T**) or false (**F**).

_____ Subgaleal hematoma can lead to rapid depletion of blood volume.

_____ Cranial CT is the optimal diagnostic tool for skull fracture.

_____ Phrenic nerve palsy may result from lateral hyperextension of the neck.

_____ Retinal hemorrhages are managed with laser therapy.

Text Reference, pages 65-71

Match the physical findings with one of the following brachial plexus injuries.

A. Duchenne Erb Palsy _____ Moro, biceps and radial reflexes are absent on the affected side

B. Klumpke's palsy _____ Hand grasp is absent

_____ Arm is adducted and internally rotated

Text Reference, page 72

CHAPTER 7

The High Risk Newborn: Anticipation, Evaluation, Management and Outcome

For the following maternal conditions or problems, identify potential neonatal complications.

UTI _____

Cigarette smoking _____

Maternal anemia _____

Bleeding _____

Text Reference, pages 76-77

Identify maternal, placental or fetal etiologies for SGA, LGA and the premature neonate.

	SGA	LGA	Premature
Maternal			
Placental			
Fetal			

Text Reference, pages 76-78

PART 2 – ASSESSMENT AND TREATMENT IN THE IMMEDIATE POSTNATAL PERIOD

Identify risks associated with the following fetal characteristics:

Oligohydramnios _____

Multiple Gestation _____

Polyhydramnios _____

Text Reference, pages 77-78

State the infant classification (preterm, late preterm) and the birth weight classification (NBW, LBW, SGA, etc.):

2500 gm, 39 weeks gestation _____

2400 gm, 31 weeks gestation _____

4300 gm, 32 weeks gestation _____

3100 gm, 41 weeks gestation _____

3200 gm, 36 weeks gestation _____

Text Reference, pages 78-79

Identify at least five common problems associated with prematurity:

1. _____
2. _____
3. _____
4. _____
5. _____

Text Reference, pages 81-82

Discuss the management of intrauterine growth restriction.

_____

_____

_____

Text Reference, pages 89-91

Discuss short and long term outcomes of SGA/IUGR infants.

_____
_____
_____
_____
_____
_____
_____

Text Reference, page 91

CHAPTER 8

Assessment of the Newborn History and Physician Examination of the Newborn

What are the normal parameters in neonatal assessment for

Skin color _____

Respiratory rate _____

Heart rate _____

Text Reference, page 98

Explain the significance of a split in the S_2 heart sound.

_____
_____
_____

Text Reference, page 98

Match the physical characteristics listed below to the following conditions.

A. Erythema toxicum

B. Milia

C. Dermal Melanocytosis

D. None

E. Sebaceous hyperplasia

_____ Appear primarily on the nose

_____ Filled with eosinophils

_____ Bluish in color

_____ Resolve within the 1st week of life

_____ Require treatment

Text Reference, page 101

PART 2 – ASSESSMENT AND TREATMENT IN THE IMMEDIATE POSTNATAL PERIOD

Describe the procedures to assess hip dislocation.

_____

_____

_____

Text Reference, page 102

Indicate if the following statements are true or false (**T** or **F**) regarding the assessment of the head, neck and mouth of the newborn.

_____ Mobility of the suture lines rules out craniosynostosis

_____ Caput succedaneum presents with a soft ping pong sensation of skull bones

_____ Epstein's pearls require topical treatment with Nystatin

_____ Cephalohematomas are the result of subperiosteal bleeding therefore they do not cross suture lines

Text Reference, pages 102-104

What etiologies should be considered when marked jitteriness is noted?

_____

_____

_____

Text Reference, page 104

Discuss newborn transition assessment.

_____

_____

_____

_____

Text Reference, page 107

CHAPTER 9

Care of the Well Newborn

Discuss family-centered maternity care.

Text Reference, page 106

Discuss routine umbilical cord care.

Text Reference, page 106

Indicate if the following statements are true (**T**) or false (**F**) regarding neonatal circumcision.

_____ Acetaminophen is an effective adjunct to analgesia.

_____ Infants with hypospadias would benefit from circumcision.

_____ Infants with chordee should not be circumcised.

_____ Local anesthetic is not necessary for the procedure.

_____ Oral intake should be restricted prior to the procedure being performed.

Text Reference, page 113

Discuss AAP's discharge criteria for late preterm infants.

Text Reference, page 115

PART 3 – GENERAL NEWBORN CONDITIONS

CHAPTER 10

Genetic Issues Presenting in the Nursery

Name three drugs that are known human teratogens.

1. _____
2. _____
3. _____

Text Reference, page 119, Table 10.1

What aspects of the prenatal and perinatal events should be evaluated?

_____
_____
_____

Text Reference, pages 121-122

Describe and differentiate the physical findings associated with Trisomy 13, Trisomy 18 and Trisomy 21.

_____
_____
_____
_____
_____

Text Reference, page 124, Table 10.2

What physical assessment finding warrants consideration of a muscle biopsy?

_____
_____

Text Reference, page 130

CHAPTER 11

Multiple Births

Review the following characteristics and **check all that apply** to multiple gestations.

- ❏ Congenital malformations risk is increased in twin gestations.

- ❏ Fetal growth patterns are similar in twin and singleton gestations until the 20th week of pregnancy.

- ❏ In twin to twin transfusion syndrome, the donor twin is anemic, hypovolemic and intrauterine growth is restricted.

- ❏ Mortality increases threefold and fourfold for triplet and quadruplet births, respectively.

Text Reference, pages 135-139

CHAPTER 12

Maternal Drug Abuse, Infant Exposure and Neonatal Abstinence Syndrome

List the most common illicit drugs abused in the United States:

1. _____
2. _____
3. _____
4. _____

Text Reference, page 141

Describe the clinical signs of withdrawal in the neonate after intrauterine exposure to the following substances:

Alcohol _____

Barbiturates _____

Diazepam _____

Text Reference, page 144

Discuss nonpharmacologic interventions for the neonate with signs of withdrawal.

_____

_____

_____

Text Reference, page 146

PART 3 – GENERAL NEWBORN CONDITIONS

Identify three drugs that are used to treat a neonate experiencing narcotic withdrawal syndrome:

1. _____
2. _____
3. _____

Text Reference, pages 146-147

Discuss management of medication therapy for neonatal withdrawal, including abstinence scoring and non-pharmacological intervention.

_____
_____
_____

Text Reference, pages 146-147

Discuss breast feeding of substance exposed infants.

_____
_____
_____

Text Reference, pages 149, 154, 155

Discuss the Neonatal Abstinence Scoring tool in relation to:

Cry _____

Feedings _____

Fever _____

Moro Reflex _____

Muscle Tone _____

Tremors _____

Text Reference, pages 150-154

CHAPTER 13
Care of the Extremely Low-Birth-Weight Infant

Indicate if the following statements are true (**T**) or false (**F**) regarding care of the extremely low-birth-weight infant.

_____ Parents are usually most concerned about long term prognosis.

_____ Maintenance of thermal status is an essential part of care.

_____ Dextrose solutions of 5 or 7.5% are usually inadequate to maintain glucose levels.

_____ 7 out of 10 ELBW infants are at risk for PDA.

_____ Blood transfusions are often necessary secondary to phlebotomy losses.

Text Reference, pages 161-169

Discuss respiratory support and the extremely low-birth-weight infant.

_____

_____

_____

Text Reference, pages 165-166

Discuss initial nutritional support in extremely low-birth-weight infants.

_____

_____

_____

Text Reference, pages 170-171

Describe signs of stress in preterm infants.

_____

_____

_____

Text Reference, pages 172-178

PART 3 – GENERAL NEWBORN CONDITIONS

Give three examples of infant self regulating behavior.

1. _____
2. _____
3. _____

Text Reference, page 178

CHAPTER 14

Developmentally Supportive Care

What is the priority for developmental supportive care?

_____
_____
_____

Discuss interventions related to the following goals of developmental support.

Support autonomic stability _____
_____

Motor system intervention _____
_____

Creating environments to cultivate state organization _____
_____

Text Reference, page 178

Discuss how the physical environment can be changed to provide developmental supportive care to the premature infant.

_____
_____

Text Reference, pages 179-181

List five developmentally supportive practices:

1. _____
2. _____
3. _____
4. _____
5. _____

Text Reference, pages 179-183

CHAPTER 15

Temperature Control

Identify at least three factors that interfere with the premature infant's ability to maintain adequate body temperature:

1. _____
2. _____
3. _____

Text Reference, pages 185-186

List the physiologic changes that occur with cold stress:

1. _____
2. _____
3. _____

Text Reference, page 186

Define neutral thermal environment.

_____

_____

_____

Text Reference, page 187

Give an example of how an infant would lose heat by:

Radiation _____

Evaporation _____

Convection _____

Conduction _____

Text Reference, page 187

PART 3 – GENERAL NEWBORN CONDITIONS

CHAPTER 16

Follow Up Care of Very Preterm and Very Low-Birth-Weight Infants

Identify if the following statements are true (**T**) or false (**F**) about follow up care of the very low-birth-weight infants.

_____ The most important cause of respiratory infection in premature infants is respiratory syncytial virus.

_____ Very low-birth-weight infants should receive their routine pediatric immunizations on the same schedule as term infants including hepatitis B vaccine.

_____ The incidence of cerebral palsy in very low-birth-weight infants is 20-25%.

_____ Hearing loss occurs in 2-11% of very low-birth-weight infants.

_____ Very low-birth-weight infants do not need to see a dentist until they are 3 years old.

Text Reference, pages 193-196

Fill in the blanks.

Developmental follow-up visits are based on _____ and _____.

Text Reference, page 200

CHAPTER 17

Neonatal Transport

Discuss the legal and regulatory issues that affect neonatal transport.

_____

_____

_____

Text Reference, pages 205-209

Discuss physiologic considerations of air transport specifically related to Dalton's Law and Boyle's Law.

_____

_____

_____

Text Reference, pages 212-213

Discuss management of an infant with suspected ductal-dependent congenital heart disease during transport.

Text Reference, page 212

CHAPTER 18
Neonatal Intensive Care Unit Discharge Planning

Identify four criteria for discharge of the healthy preterm infant:

1. _____
2. _____
3. _____
4. _____

Text Reference, pages 214-215

Identify the four central tenets of Family Centered Care:

1. _____
2. _____
3. _____
4. _____

Text Reference, page 221

Identify at least three topics of discharge education that all NICU parents or caregivers need:

1. _____
2. _____
3. _____

Text Reference, page 222-223

PART 3 – GENERAL NEWBORN CONDITIONS

Discuss why a family assessment is important and list five important questions that should be asked/addressed.

1. _____
2. _____
3. _____
4. _____
5. _____

Text Reference, pages 224-225

CHAPTER 19

Decision-Making and Ethical Dilemmas

What ethical principles must be considered in the decision making process in the NICU?

_____
_____
_____

Text Reference, page 235

Discuss the approach for developing a process for ethical decision making.

_____
_____
_____

Text Reference, pages 236-238

What role should data play in ethical decision making?

_____
_____
_____

Text Reference, page 239

When should the hospital ethics committee become involved with ethical decision making in the NICU?

Text Reference, page 240

CHAPTER 20

Management of Neonatal End of Life Care & Bereavement Follow Up

Discuss the coordination of end of life care incorporating the seven key end of life domains.

1.
2.
3.
4.
5.
6.
7.

Text Reference, page 243

What are the recommendations for staff regarding provision of support to a family where life support is being withdrawn from their child?

Text Reference, page 244

PART 4 – FLUID ELECTROLYTES, NUTRITION, GASTROINTESTINAL & RENAL ISSUES

CHAPTER 21

Nutrition

Name indications for initiating parenteral nutrition.

1. _____
2. _____
3. _____

Text Reference, page 260

Describe the issues to be considered when deciding between peripheral and central PN.

_____
_____
_____

Text Reference, page 260

Discuss the glucose needs of preterm neonate.

_____
_____
_____

Text Reference, pages 260-261

Three signs of glucose intolerance include _____ and _____

with _____.

Text Reference, page 261

Identify if the following statements are true (**T**) or false (**F**) about electrolytes, vitamins and trace elements in PN feedings.

_____ The amount of calcium and phosphorus that can be administered by IV is limited by the precipitation of calcium phosphate.

_____ Copper and manganese should be withheld in PN feedings for infants with cholestatic liver disease.

_____ Carnitine is not routinely added to PN but should be considered with infants requiring long-term PN.

_____ Three-in-one PN solutions are used with neonates.

Text Reference, pages 263-267

Identify three potential complications of parenteral nutrition:

1. _____

2. _____

3. _____

Text Reference, pages 265-266

List three benefits of trophic feedings:

1. _____

2. _____

3. _____

Text Reference, page 268

List criteria that would make a neonate a candidate for transpyloric feedings:

1. _____

2. _____

3. _____

Text Reference, page 278

Match the type of infant formula with the condition that would be addressed by its use.
(an answer may apply to more than one condition)

A. Semi-elemental formula containing reduced LCT with MCT	_____	Gastroesophageal reflux
B. Extensively hydrolyzed protein	_____	Cystic fibrosis
C. Standard formula	_____	Cow's milk protein allergy
D. Significantly reduced LCT with supplemental MCT	_____	Renal insufficiency
	_____	Chylothorax

Text Reference, page 276, Table 21.7

PART 4 – FLUID ELECTROLYTES, NUTRITION, GASTROINTESTINAL & RENAL ISSUES

Discuss transition from tube feedings to breast/bottle feedings.

Text Reference, page 278

Describe the nutritional management for infants with:

NEC

Text Reference, pages 280-281

Bronchopulmonary Dysplasia

Text Reference, page 281

CHAPTER 22
Breastfeeding and Maternal Medications

Discuss the general principles/recommendations for breastfeeding healthy term infants.

Text Reference, pages 285-286

Match the following potential breastfeeding problems with the statement/phrase below.

A. Nipple trauma	_____ Common cause is incorrect infant positioning

B. Engorgement	_____ Manifests with flu like symptoms

C. Nipple soreness	_____ Onset is usually 3-5 days postpartum

D. Plugged ducts	_____ Often occurs when feeding or pumping is missed or delayed

E. Mastitis	_____ Is normal

Text Reference, pages 287-288

Indicate if the following statements are true or false (**T**) or (**F**) regarding the care and handling of breast milk.

_____ Sterilize pump parts once a week.

_____ Milk expression and storage technique can affect the composition and bacterial content of the breast milk.

_____ At the end of the second postpartum week the target daily milk volume is 500 ml.

_____ Mothers should scrub under their fingernails prior to each milk expression.

Text Reference, page 290

Indicate if breastfeeding is permissible (**P**) or not recommended (**NR**) In the following situation.

The mother has:

_____ HIV infection

_____ Hepatitis B

_____ CMV

_____ Hepatitis C

Text Reference, page 291

CHAPTER 23

Fluid & Electrolyte Management

Define TBW and discuss perinatal changes in TBW in both the term and preterm infant.

_____

_____

_____

_____

Text Reference, pages 296-297

PART 4 – FLUID ELECTROLYTES, NUTRITION, GASTROINTESTINAL & RENAL ISSUES

Discuss sources of water loss in the premature infant.

Text Reference, page 297

Describe the effect of insensible water loss on the very low-birth-weight infant.

Text Reference, pages 297-298

Identify at least two predisposing factors to dehydration:

1. _____
2. _____

Text Reference, page 300

What are the physical signs and symptoms of dehydration?

Text Reference, page 300

Describe and differentiate hyponatremia due to ECF volume depletion, normal ECF volume and ECF volume excess.

Text Reference, pages 301-302

Discuss the administration of a fluid challenge in managing oliguria.

_____

_____

_____

Text Reference, pages 303-305

Identify whether the following causes of oliguria are due to prerenal (**PR**), parenchymal (**P**) or postrenal (**POR**) causes.

_____ Decreased preload

_____ Posterior urethral valves

_____ DIC

_____ Acute tubular necrosis

_____ Increased peripheral resistance

_____ Uric acid nephropathy

Text Reference, page 304, Table 23.4

Match the condition with one of the following findings:

A. Metabolic acidosis with anion gap > 15 mEq/L

B. Metabolic acidosis with anion gap < 15 mEq/L

C. Metabolic alkalosis (low urinary chloride)

D. Metabolic alkalosis (high urinary chloride)

_____ Inborn errors of metabolism

_____ Diarrhea

_____ Nasogastric suction

_____ Acute renal failure

_____ Small bowel drainage

_____ Hypokalemia

_____ Massive blood product transfusion

Text Reference, pages 305-307

List three complications of hypokalemia:

1. _____

2. _____

3. _____

Text Reference, page 307

PART 4 – FLUID ELECTROLYTES, NUTRITION, GASTROINTESTINAL & RENAL ISSUES

List three predisposing factors to hyperkalemia:

1. _____
2. _____
3. _____

Text Reference, pages 307-308

What are the three pharmacologic therapies used to treat hyperkalemia?

1. _____
2. _____
3. _____

Text Reference, pages 308-309

Discuss the management of the infant with severe chronic lung disease requiring diuretic therapy.

_____
_____
_____

Text Reference, page 311

CHAPTER 24

Hypoglycemia & Hyperglycemia

Define hypoglycemia in the newborn.

_____
_____
_____

Text Reference, pages 313-314

Explain each of the following etiologies of hypoglycemia.

Hyperinsulinemic hypoglycemia _____

_____

Large for gestational age _____

_____

Decreased production / stores _____

_____

Increased utilization and/or decreased production _____

_____

Text Reference, pages 314-315

Describe the clinical signs and symptoms of hypoglycemia.

_____

_____

_____

Text Reference, page 316

Discuss possible mechanisms of action related to maternal/infant therapy with beta blockers (labetalol or propanolol).

_____

_____

_____

Text Reference, page 315

Indicate management of hypoglycemia for asymptomatic infants at risk for hypoglycemia.

_____

_____

_____

Text Reference, page 313

SECTION 4 – FLUID ELECTROLYTES, NUTRITION, GASTROINTESTINAL & RENAL ISSUES

Indicate management for hypoglycemia for infants who are symptomatic.

Text Reference, page 313

Identify at least three differential diagnoses for hypoglycemia:

1.
2.
3.

Text Reference, page 317

Name four indications for IV glucose therapy.

1.
2.
3.
4.

Text Reference, page 318

Describe when glucagon should be given.

Text Reference, page 321

Identify at least four etiologies of hyperglycemia:

1. _____
2. _____
3. _____
4. _____

Text Reference, pages 322-323

Explain why when an infant is given insulin, it is prudent to decrease the glucose levels slowly.

_____

_____

_____

Text Reference, pages 323-324

CHAPTER 25

Abnormalities of Serum Calcium and Magnesium

Fill in the blanks.

Calcium ions in _____ and _____

are essential for many biochemical processes.

Text Reference, page 326

Describe the homeostasis function of the following hormones:

1. PTH _____
2. Calcitriol _____
3. Vitamin D _____

Text Reference, pages 326-327

Indicate the statements that are **true** about postnatal changes in serum calcium concentrations.

- ❏ At birth, umbilical serum calcium level is elevated.
- ❏ In healthy babies, calcium concentrations decline for the first 24-48 hours.
- ❏ Serum calcium concentrations in the first three days are inversely correlated with gestational age.
- ❏ Calcium levels reach their highest level at 2 days of age.

Text Reference, page 328

PART 4 – FLUID ELECTROLYTES, NUTRITION, GASTROINTESTINAL & RENAL ISSUES

Identify three likely components of the infant's history in cases of late onset hypocalcemia:

1. _____
2. _____
3. _____

Text Reference, page 328

Describe the clinical presentation of early onset hypocalcemia in preterm infants.

_____

_____

_____

Text Reference, page 328

Identify at least three risks of therapy with calcium:

1. _____
2. _____
3. _____

Text Reference, page 329

Identify three etiologies of hypercalcemia:

1. _____
2. _____
3. _____

Text Reference, page 331

Check **all** the symptoms listed that are consistent with hypercalcemia.

- ❏ Vomiting
- ❏ Hypotension
- ❏ Enlarged spleen and liver
- ❏ Arrhythmias
- ❏ Polyuria

Text Reference, pages 331-333

What is the best treatment for hypercalcemia due to hypervitaminosis A and D?

- ❏ Calcitonin
- ❏ Glucocorticoids
- ❏ Inorganic phosphate

Text Reference, page 333

Name three causes of hypermagnesemia.

1. _____
2. _____
3. _____

Text Reference, page 333

When hypermagnesemia is severe which of the following are the best treatments.

- ❏ calcium infusion via central line
- ❏ removal of source of exogenous magnesium
- ❏ exchange transfusion

Text Reference, pages 333-334

PART 4 – FLUID ELECTROLYTES, NUTRITION, GASTROINTESTINAL & RENAL ISSUES

CHAPTER 26

Neonatal Hyperbilirubinemia

Identify which of the following statements regarding bilirubin are true.

- ❏ Bilirubin is fat soluble.
- ❏ Bilirubin bound to albumin crosses the blood brain barrier.
- ❏ The toxicity of bilirubin is not affected by acidosis.
- ❏ Bilirubin binds to albumin and travels to the liver.

Text Reference, page 336

What drug displaces bilirubin from albumin.

_____

Text Reference, page 336

Describe nonpathologic hyperbilirubinemia in terms of levels of bilirubin and the age of the infant.

_____
_____
_____

Text Reference, page 337

Name five characteristics of hyperbilirubinemia.

1. _____
2. _____
3. _____
4. _____
5. _____

Text Reference, page 337

Describe the clinical presentation of breast milk jaundice and highlight how it is different from nonphysiologic jaundice.

_____
_____
_____

Text Reference, page 340

List four contribution factors associated with hyperbilirubinemia:

1. _____
2. _____
3. _____
4. _____

Text Reference, page 342

Discuss the physical assessment techniques used to detect jaundice.

_____
_____
_____

Text Reference, pages 342-343

Discuss when direct or conjugated bilirubin should be measured.

_____
_____
_____

Text Reference, page 343

Identify the clinical tests that should be initiated in cases of nonphysiologic jaundice and their purpose.

_____
_____
_____

Text Reference, page 343

True (**T**) or False (**F**)

_____ The hour-specific total bilirubin guidelines published by the AAP can be used for initiation of therapy for babies less than 34 weeks gestation.

Test Reference, page 344

PART 4 – FLUID ELECTROLYTES, NUTRITION, GASTROINTESTINAL & RENAL ISSUES

Identify the steps in management of unconjugated hyperbilirubinemia:

1. _____
2. _____
3. _____

Text Reference, pages 344-346

List five risk factors for hyperbilirubinemia neurotoxicity:

1. _____
2. _____
3. _____
4. _____
5. _____

Text Reference, page 345

Explain how phototherapy works.

_____
_____
_____

Text Reference, pages 345-346

What types of lights are most efficient for phototherapy?

_____
_____

Text Reference, page 346

List three adverse effects of phototherapy:

1. _____
2. _____
3. _____

Text Reference, page 347

Discuss exchange transfusion in the treatment of hyperbilirubinemia, including indications, blood type & volume used, transfusion technique and follow-up.

_____

_____

_____

Text Reference, pages 347-349

List at least three complications of exchange transfusion:

1. _____

2. _____

3. _____

Text Reference, page 349

A neonate has a direct bilirubin level of 2.2 mg/dL. What is the next step?

_____ initiate work up to determine underlying cause

_____ place the infant under continuous phototherapy

_____ prepare for exchange transfusion

Test Reference, page 350

Define kernicterus.

_____

_____

_____

Text Reference, pages 349-350

List four disorders that cause neonatal cholestasis:

1. _____

2. _____

3. _____

4. _____

Text Reference, pages 350-351

PART 4 – FLUID ELECTROLYTES, NUTRITION, GASTROINTESTINAL & RENAL ISSUES

Discuss management of parenteral nutrition (PN) associated cholestasis.

_____

_____

_____

Text Reference, page 351

CHAPTER 27

Necrotizing Entercolitis

Which of the following statements are true (**T**) or false (**F**) regarding necrotizing enterocolitis?

_____ Male infants are at increased risk for developing this disease.

_____ Prematurity is the single greatest risk factor.

_____ Infants exposed to cocaine have an increased risk for developing the disease.

_____ Prolonged empiric antimicrobial use has not been associated with NEC occurrence.

Text Reference, page 354

Approximately _____ % of infants with NEC are term.

Text Reference, page 354

Identify the clinical findings of NEC.

_____

_____

_____

Text Reference, pages 356-357

Explain the Bell staging criteria.

_____

_____

_____

Text Reference, page 357

Discuss possible differential diagnoses for NEC.

_____
_____
_____

Text Reference, page 358

Discuss the medical management of NEC.

_____
_____
_____

Text Reference, pages 359-362

Describe the typical x-ray findings associated with NEC.

_____
_____
_____

Text Reference, page 359

Identify two indications for surgical intervention with NEC:

1. _____
2. _____

Text Reference, pages 362-363

Discuss the prognosis and preventive measures.

_____
_____
_____

Text Reference, pages 363-364

PART 4 – FLUID ELECTROLYTES, NUTRITION, GASTROINTESTINAL & RENAL ISSUES

CHAPTER 28

Neonatal Kidney Conditions

Indicate which of the following statements about functional renal development are true (**T**) or false (**F**).

_____ GFR increases parallel with body and kidney growth.

_____ Increased GFR is responsible for the limited ability of premature infants to excrete large potassium loads.

_____ Bicarbonate handling is limited by the neonate's low bicarbonate threshold.

_____ The newborn has a limited ability to dilute urine.

_____ Tubular resorption of sodium in the fetus is low until the 24th week of gestation.

Text Reference, pages 368-369

Assessment of renal function of the neonate is based on what three parameters?

1. _____

2. _____

3. _____

Text Reference, pages 370-371

In interpreting renal function test, which of the following statements are true (**T**) or false (**F**).

_____ Full term infants have a limited urine concentrating ability

_____ Protein excretion is similar in both premature and term infants

_____ Presence of the hematuria is common and often benign

_____ Hyaline and fine granular casts are common in dehydration

Text Reference, pages 372 & 376

_____ is the most reliable method of urine sampling

for diagnosis of urinary tract infection.

Text Reference, page 377

Discuss the following lab values in regard to evaluation of neonatal renal function.

Serum creatinine _____

_____

BUN _____

_____

Text Reference, page 377

Indicate the purpose of each of the radiological studies in evaluating neonatal renal status.

Ultrasound _____

Voiding cystourethography _____

Radionuclide scintigraphy _____

Text Reference, pages 378-380

Define the causes of:

Prerenal azotemia _____

Intrinsic acute kidney injury _____

Postrenal acute kidney injury _____

Text Reference, page 381-383

Discuss how acute kidney injury is managed in the neonate.

_____

_____

_____

Text Reference, pages 383-386

PART 4 – FLUID ELECTROLYTES, NUTRITION, GASTROINTESTINAL & RENAL ISSUES

Identify three renal causes of neonatal hypertension:

1. _____
2. _____
3. _____

Text Reference, pages 388-393

Identify four predisposing factors to renal vein thrombosis:

1. _____
2. _____
3. _____
4. _____

Text Reference, page 393

Identify three renal causes of hematuria:

1. _____
2. _____
3. _____

Text Reference, pages 396-397

What medical conditions would contraindicate circumcision in the neonate?

_____
_____
_____

Text Reference, pages 397-398

Define renal tubular acidosis.

Text Reference, pages 398-399

What is the treatment for renal tubular necrosis (RTA), including distal, proximal and hyperkalemic RTA?

Text Reference, page 399

How is nephrocalcinosis detected?

Text Reference, page 399

PART 5 – RESPIRATORY DISORDERS

CHAPTER 29

Mechanical Ventilation

Regarding CPAP:

Identify three disadvantages with the use of CPAP:

1. _____
2. _____
3. _____

Text Reference, pages 401-402

What is now commonly used as an alternative to CPAP? Describe the treatment, advantages, and disadvantages.

_____
_____
_____

Text Reference, page 402-403

Describe synchronized and patient-triggered ventilators in the care of neonates, including advantages and disadvantages.

_____
_____
_____

Text Reference, page 403-404

What are the general characteristics of volume targeted ventilators?

_____
_____
_____

Text Reference, page 405

List three types of high frequency ventilators:

1. _____

2. _____

3. _____

Text Reference, page 405

Describe high frequency ventilators, including characteristics, advantages, disadvantages, and indications.

_____

_____

_____

Text Reference, pages 405-406

Fill in the blanks.

In regard to how ventilator changes affect blood gases:

Which parameter can you increase to give you the greatest rise in PaO_2? _____

Discuss the difference in MAP required for infants with severe respiratory distress syndrome compared to the MAP sufficient for infants with normal lungs.

_____

_____

CO_2 elimination depends on _____ .

Text Reference, pages 407-410

Define the following terms.

Compliance _____

_____

Functional residual capacity _____

_____

Work of breathing _____

_____

V/Q matching _____

_____

Text Reference, page 411

PART 5 – RESPIRATORY DISORDERS

Indicate if the following statements/phrases are true (**T**) or false (**F**) about mechanical ventilation for neonates with meconium aspiration.

_____ The positive pressure may result in pneumothorax

_____ Low levels of PEEP are useful

_____ Use of patient-triggered ventilation should be avoided.

_____ Frequencies higher than 10 Hz should be used if high frequency ventilation is initiated

Text Reference, pages 415-416

List adjunct therapy to use in conjunction with mechanical ventilation:

1. _____
2. _____
3. _____

Text Reference, pages 417-418

List the four categories of complications that are associated with mechanical ventilation and list one example of each:

1. _____
2. _____
3. _____
4. _____

Text Reference, page 418

CHAPTER 30

Blood Gas and Pulmonary Function Monitoring

What information does arterial blood gas measurement provide?

_____

_____

_____

Text Reference, pages 419-420

How does the pulse oximeter work?

Text Reference, pages 420-421

Discuss the use of transcutaneous CO_2 monitoring.

Text Reference, page 422-424

CHAPTER 31

Apnea

Check all of the following statements/phrases that are **true** about apnea.

❏ Obstructive apnea occurs even though inspiratory efforts persist

❏ The incidence of apnea is similar in both premature and term neonates

❏ Infants may not respond to tactile stimulation

❏ A history of apnea increases the risk of SIDS

❏ Caffeine is the drug of choice

❏ Specific therapy should be directed toward the underlying cause

Text Reference, pages 426-431

CHAPTER 32

Transient Tachypnea of the Newborn

Check **all** of the following statements or phrases that are **true** about transient tachypnea of the newborn.

❏ Predisposing factors include precipitous delivery or cesarean delivery

❏ It is usually a benign, self-limiting process

❏ Differential diagnoses include meconium aspiration

❏ It is a disease more common to males

❏ Oxygen is the primary treatment

Text Reference, pages 432-433

PART 5 – RESPIRATORY DISORDERS

CHAPTER 33

Respiratory Distress Syndrome

The primary cause of respiratory distress syndrome is _____.

Text Reference, page 436

Describe the tests used to assess fetal lung maturity.

_____

_____

Text Reference, pages 437-438

Discuss the physiologic maneuvers that neonates with RDS use to establish Functional Residual Capacity (FRC) and optimize gas exchange.

_____

_____

_____

Text Reference, page 438

List four differential diagnoses for respiratory distress syndrome:

1. _____
2. _____
3. _____
4. _____

Text Reference, page 439

Discuss steps to take when weaning infants with RDS from CPAP.

_____

_____

_____

Text Reference, page 441

List four complications of CPAP:

1. _____
2. _____
3. _____
4. _____

Text Reference, pages 441-442

Indicate if the following statements about surfactant replacement therapy are true (**T**) or false (**F**).

_____ Repeat doses of surfactant may be needed to achieve a therapeutic response.

_____ Pulmonary hemorrhage is increased in neonates who have a PDA.

_____ Four doses of Survanta may be given.

_____ High FiO_2 levels are required for optimization of functional residual capacity.

Text Reference, pages 442-444

Identify the three acute complications that occur with the administration of exogenous surfactant therapy:

1. _____
2. _____
3. _____

Text Reference, page 444

Discuss volume-limited, time-cycled ventilation in relation to RDS and surfactant administration.

_____
_____
_____

Text Reference, page 445

PART 5 – RESPIRATORY DISORDERS

CHAPTER 34

Bronchopulmonary Dysplasia/Chronic Lung Disease

Check **all** of the following statements that are **true** about chronic lung disease.

❏ Acute lung injury is caused by prolonged exposure to oxygen and barotrauma from the mechanical ventilation.

❏ Surfactant therapy has significantly reduced the number of infants who progress to chronic lung disease.

❏ Mortality is 25% during the first year of life.

❏ Neonates are at increased risk for childhood asthma.

Text Reference, pages 448-459

List five associated complications of Bronchopulmonary Dysplasia (BPD):

1. _____
2. _____
3. _____
4. _____
5. _____

Text Reference, pages 456-458

CHAPTER 35

Meconium Aspiration

Check **all** of the following statements that are **true** about meconium aspiration.

❏ Broad-spectrum antibiotics are usually given to infants with meconium aspiration.

❏ It occurs more frequently in term and post term neonates.

❏ Fetal stress is a major contributory factor.

❏ Adequate airway management can prevent meconium aspiration.

❏ There is a 10-20% incidence of pneumothorax.

Text Reference, pages 461-466

Discuss the use of surfactant in meconium aspiration syndrome.

_____

_____

_____

Text Reference, page 465

CHAPTER 36

Persistent Pulmonary Hypertension of the Newborn

What is the pathophysiology involved with persistent pulmonary hypertension?

_____

_____

_____

Text Reference, pages 467-470

Identify at least three perinatal risk factors for persistent pulmonary hypertension of the newborn:

1. _____

2. _____

3. _____

Text Reference, page 468

Discuss the management approaches for treating persistent pulmonary hypertension of the newborn.

_____

_____

_____

Text Reference, pages 471-477

Describe the mechanism of action of nitric oxide in treatment of persistent pulmonary hypertension.

_____

_____

_____

Text Reference, pages 472-473

Discuss the use of complementary pharmacological therapies in management of persistent pulmonary hypertension.

_____

_____

_____

Text Reference, page 474-477

PART 5 – RESPIRATORY DISORDERS

The availability of what two therapies led to the reduction of PPHN-associated mortality?

1. _____

2. _____

Text Reference, page 477

CHAPTER 37

Pulmonary Hemorrhage

Check **all** of the following statements or phrases that are **true** about pulmonary hemorrhage.

❏ Sudden cardiorespiratory decompensation is common

❏ Pulmonary edema is a common long term complication

❏ Pathophysiology is unclear

❏ There is a high death rate

Text Reference, pages 478-481

Discuss the treatment of pulmonary hemorrhage.

_____

_____

_____

Text Reference, page 480

CHAPTER 38

Pulmonary Air Leak

Describe the clinical presentation of a pneumothorax.

_____

_____

_____

Text Reference, page 483

Describe the x-ray findings consistent with a pneumothorax.

Text Reference, page 484

What is the purpose of transillumination in diagnosing a pneumothorax?

Text Reference, page 484

When is needle aspiration indicated in treatment of pneumothorax?

Text Reference, page 484

Discuss the treatment of Pulmonary Interstitial Emphysema (PIE).

Text Reference, pages 487-488

True (**T**) or False (**F**)

_____ Pneumopericardium is a common cause of cardiac tamponade.

Test Reference, pages 487-488

PART 5 – RESPIRATORY DISORDERS

CHAPTER 39

Extracorporeal Membrane Oxygenation

Identify the clinical indication(s) for ECMO.

_____
_____

Text Reference, page 491-493

Define oxygenation index (OI) and how it relates to meeting ECMO criteria.

_____
_____
_____
_____
_____

Text Reference, page 491

Indicate at least three contraindications for ECMO therapy.

1. _____
2. _____
3. _____

Text Reference, pages 493

Describe the difference between venovenous ECMO support and venoarterial ECMO support and the indications for each.

_____
_____
_____

Text Reference, page 493-494

Discuss the cardiovascular complications of ECMO.

Text Reference, page 499

Discuss survival and neurodevelopmental outcomes for ECMO patients.

Text Reference, pages 500-501

PART 6 – CARDIOVASCULAR DISORDERS

CHAPTER 40

Shock

Define shock.

_____

_____

_____

Text Reference, page 502

Identify and define the five primary causes of neonatal shock:

1. _____
2. _____
3. _____
4. _____
5. _____

Text Reference, page 502-504

Describe the pathophysiology of circulatory failure as it relates to:

Hypovolemic shock _____

_____

Distributive shock _____

_____

Cardiogenic shock _____

_____

Obstructive shock _____

_____

Text Reference, pages 503-504

Compare compensated and uncompensated shock.

Compensated: _____

_____

Uncompensated: _____

_____

Text Reference, page 504

Discuss shock and its management as it relates to the very low birth weight neonate in the immediate postnatal period.

_____

_____

_____

Text Reference, page 507

Discuss shock and its management as it relates to the preterm neonate with Patent Ductus Arteriosus (PDA).

_____

_____

_____

Text Reference, page 508

Match the drug with its effect in treating shock.

A. Hydrocortisone

B. Dopamine

C. Dobutamine

D. Epinephrine

E. Calcium Gluconate (10%)

_____ Inotropic effects are independent of norepinephrine stores

_____ Increases myocardial contractility and peripheral vascular resistance; may be effective in patients who do not respond to Dopamine

_____ Increases renal mesenteric and coronary blood flow with little effect on cardiac output at low doses

_____ Used to treat hypotension refractory to volume expansion

_____ May be necessary if infant has received large amounts of volume replacement

Text Reference, pages 505-507

PART 6 – CARDIOVASCULAR DISORDERS

CHAPTER 41

Cardiac Disorders

Discuss the three factors that determine the timing of presentation and accompanying symptomatology of congenital heart disease (CHD) in the newborn.

_____
_____
_____

Text Reference, page 512

Check **all** that describe the most common symptoms of CHD in the first few weeks of life.

- ❏ Cyanosis
- ❏ Asymptomatic heart murmur
- ❏ Bradycardia
- ❏ Arrhythmia

Text Reference, pages 514-519

The degree of visible cyanosis depends on what two variables?

1. _____
2. _____

Text Reference, pages 514-515

Discuss how these two variables affect the clinical presentation of cyanosis.

_____
_____
_____

Text Reference, page 514-515

Identify at least two pulmonary disorders that may result in cyanosis:

1. _____
2. _____

Text Reference, page 515

Identify two conditions when cyanosis may occur in an infant without hypoxemia:

1. _____

2. _____

Text Reference, page 515

Identify which of the following statements are correct regarding congestive heart failure (CHF).

❏ CHF is a clinical diagnosis made based primarily on a set of symptoms.

❏ The diagnosis of CHF is dependent on specific radiological and/or laboratory findings.

❏ The symptoms of CHF are related to the compensatory attempts of the body to improve circulation.

❏ CHF is directly related to the amount of oxygen in the blood.

❏ CHF occurs when the heart is unable to meet the metabolic demands of the tissues.

Text Reference, page 515

List at least three signs and symptoms of congestive heart failure:

1. _____

2. _____

3. _____

Text Reference, page 515

What two factors related to heart murmurs provide important clues to the nature of the heart defect in the neonate?

1. _____

2. _____

Text Reference, pages 517-519

When is the recommended timing for fetal echocardiography for prenatal diagnosis of congenital heart disease?

_____

_____

_____

Text Reference, pages 519-521

PART 6 – CARDIOVASCULAR DISORDERS

Name at least two indications for fetal echocardiography relative to:

Fetal Risk Factors

1. _____
2. _____

Text Reference, page 520

Maternal Risk Factors

1. _____
2. _____

Text Reference, page 520

Family Related Indications

1. _____
2. _____

Text Reference, pages 520-521

Describe specific physical characteristics that should be assessed carefully when performing a physical examination on the neonate with congenital heart disease.

_____
_____
_____

Text Reference, page 521-522

What specific physical finding is significant because it suggests coarctation of the aorta?

_____

Text Reference, page 522

Name at least three cardiac anomalies that are commonly associated with specific chromosomal syndromes.

1. _____
2. _____
3. _____

Text Reference, pages 523-525

Regarding chest x-ray findings relative to congenital heart disease, answer the following:

Why may it be difficult to determine the size of the neonatal heart?

Why is it significant to note dextrocardia and situs inversus?

What do dark lung fields suggest?

What do diffusely opaque lung fields suggest?

Text Reference, page 526

Why is the neonatal ECG not a reliable indicator of congenital heart disease?

Text Reference, page 526

What determinations should be made when interpreting a neonatal ECG?

Text Reference, page 526

When an ECG is abnormal, how can incorrect lead placement be ruled out?

Text Reference, page 526

PART 6 – CARDIOVASCULAR DISORDERS

What single test is the most sensitive and specific tool in the initial evaluation of the neonate suspected of having congenital heart disease? Describe how to perform this test.

_____

_____

_____

Text Reference, pages 526-530

Name two indications for initiating a PGE_1 infusion.

1. _____

2. _____

Which lesions may be made worse with PGE_1 therapy?

_____

_____

_____

What are the most significant side effects of PGE_1 infusion?

_____

_____

_____

Text Reference, pages 530-531

Why is it appropriate to begin PGE_1 infusion on an infant who presents with shock and who is suspected of having a ductal-dependent heart lesion before a definitive diagnosis can be made?

_____

_____

_____

Text Reference, pages 530-531

Describe care of the infant receiving PGE₁ infusion, including the following:

Airway maintenance _____

_____

Vascular access _____

_____

Monitoring vital signs and arterial blood gases _____

_____

Text Reference, pages 530-531

Compare and contrast the action of dopamine and dobutamine for treating cardiac patients.

_____

_____

_____

Text Reference, pages 531-532

What non-invasive test can provide information about the structure and function of the heart? What are concerns that should be addressed during the testing procedure?

_____

_____

_____

Text Reference, page 532

Name three indications for the use of cardiac catheterization.

1. _____

2. _____

3. _____

Text Reference, pages 532-534

PART 6 – CARDIOVASCULAR DISORDERS

Match the type of heart lesions/problem with the disease entities:

a. Left sided obstructive lesions
   /Ductal dependent systemic blood flow

b. Duct dependent pulmonary blood flow

c. Parallel circulation

d. Intracardiac mixing

e. Left to right shunt lesions

_____ Coarctation of the aorta

_____ Pulmonary atresia

_____ Ebstein's anomaly

_____ Transposition of the great arteries

_____ Patent ductus arteriosus

_____ Hypoplastic left heart syndrome

_____ Tetralogy of Fallot

_____ Ventricular septal defect

_____ Total Anomalous Pulmonary Venous Connection

_____ Truncus arteriosus

Text Reference Pages 535-558

Complete the following statements.

In hypoplastic left heart syndrome, constriction of the ductus arteriosus leads to _____.

Text Reference, pages 540-542

In duct dependent pulmonary flow lesions, closure of the ductus arteriosus results in _____.

Text Reference, page 542

Name three anatomic or hemodynamic findings of pulmonary valve stenosis.

1. _____
2. _____
3. _____

Text Reference, page 543

In a neonate with tricuspid atresia, the immediate medical management is primarily aimed at maintenance of _____.

Text Reference, pages 545-547

Discuss the hemodynamic findings of:

Pulmonary atresia with intact ventricular septum

Text Reference, pages 544-545

Tricuspid atresia

Text Reference, pages 545-547

Tetralogy of Fallot

Text Reference, pages 547-549

Ebstein's anomaly

Text Reference, pages 548-549

Transposition of the great arteries

Text Reference, pages 549-551

PART 6 – CARDIOVASCULAR DISORDERS

Truncus arteriosus

Text Reference, page 551

Total anomalous pulmonary venous connection

Text Reference, pages 551-553

Describe the typical presentation of a neonate with patent ductus arteriosus.

Text Reference, pages 554-555

Identify the initial management strategies for treatment of patent ductus arteriosus.

Text Reference, page 555

What is a common electrocardiogram finding in a neonate with a complete atrioventricular canal?

Text Reference, page 555

What cardiac anomaly is the most common cause of congestive heart failure after the initial neonatal period?

- ❏ Coarctation of aorta
- ❏ Truscipid of arteriosus
- ❏ Ventricular septal defect

Text Reference, page 556

Complete the statements below.

Ventricular septal detects are classified by _____.

The diagnosis of ventricular septal defect is confirmed by _____

Text Reference, pages 556-557

Identify three types of acquired heart disease:

1. _____
2. _____
3. _____

Text Reference, page 562

Check **all** of the following statements that are true about acquired heart disease.

- ❏ Myocarditis is an isolated entity.
- ❏ Perinatal asphyxia is a predisposing factor for transient myocardial ischemia.
- ❏ The most common hypertrophic cardiomyopathy occurs in infants of diabetic mothers
- ❏ Acute myocardrtis can be fatal

Text Reference, page 562

PART 6 – CARDIOVASCULAR DISORDERS

Describe the characteristics of the following vasodilators in treatment of cardiac disease.

Sodium nitroprusside _____

_____

Nitroglycerin _____

_____

Hydralazine _____

_____

Enalapril _____

_____

Text Reference, pages 565

Describe the characteristics of the following vasodilators in treatment of cardiac disease.

Beta blockers (Propranolol)_____

_____

Calcium channel blockers (Verapamil) _____

_____

Text Reference, page 565

Compare initial doses with maintenance doses of digoxin.

_____

_____

Text Reference, pages 565-566

Identify three signs of toxicity of digoxin:

1. _____
2. _____
3. _____

Text Reference, page 566

Describe management of digoxin toxicity.

_____

_____

_____

Text Reference, page 566

Check **all** of the following statements that are **true** about furosemide.

_____ The recommended starting dose is 1-2 mg per dose.

_____ It takes approximately four hours to see diuresis occur.

_____ If no response occurs, a loop diuretic should be added.

_____ Chronic use can lead to urinary tract stones.

_____ Calcium levels should be monitored during therapy.

_____ When doses are changed from parenteral to oral doses, the dose should be decreased.

_____ Furosemide should not be given if an aminoglycoside is also being given.

Text Reference, pages 566-567

What is a complication of combination diuretic therapy?

_____

_____

_____

Text Reference, pages 566-567

Identify three broad categories of arrhythmias in neonates:

1. _____

2. _____

3. _____

Text Reference, page 567

PART 6 – CARDIOVASCULAR DISORDERS

Match the statements or phrases with the listed neonatal arrhythmias. **More than one answer may apply.**

a. Supraventricular tachychardia

b. Complete heart block

c. Ventricular fibrillation

d. Ventricular tachycardia

e. Sinus bradycardia

f. Sinus tachycardia

g. First degree artrioventricular block

h. Second degree artrioventricular block

j. Premature atrial contractions

k. Premature ventricular contractions

_____ It is a rare arrhythmia in neonates

_____ Occurs during sleep or vagal maneuvers

_____ Most common symptomatic arrhythmia in children

_____ It is almost always an agonal preterminal arrhythmia

_____ Refers to the absence of conduction of any atrial activity to the ventricles

_____ Treatment is based on the underlying cause

_____ PR interval is longer than 0.15 seconds

_____ Rate is greater than 200 beats per min

_____ May occur with supraventricular tachycardia

_____ Are wide QRS complex beats

_____ Treated with lidocaine

_____ Digoxin is the initial therapy

Text Reference, pages 567, 569-571

What has become the "drug of choice" for acute management of tachycardia? _____

Describe the action of this medication.

_____

_____

_____

Text Reference, page 573

PART 7 – HEMATOLOGIC DISORDERS

CHAPTER 42

Blood Products Used in the Newborns

Name three reasons why directed or designated donor blood is **not** recommended for neonatal transfusion.

1. _____
2. _____

Text Reference, page 577

Identify four benefits of leukoreduction of blood products:

1. _____
2. _____
3. _____
4. _____

Text Reference, page 577-578

Discuss transfusion-associated graft-versus-host disease (TA-GVHD). Identify those neonates at risk and how it can be prevented.

_____
_____
_____

Text Reference, pages 578, 581

List two indications for neonatal packed red blood cell transfusion:

1. _____
2. _____

Text Reference, page 579

PART 7 – HEMATOLOGIC DISORDERS

List six potential side effects of red cell transfusion including the cause and significant symptoms of each:

1. _____

2. _____

3. _____

4. _____

5. _____

6. _____

Text Reference, pages 580-581

Identify the primary indication for neonatal fresh frozen plasma (FFP) infusion.

_____

Text Reference, page 581

Name two conditions where FFP is **not** recommended and explain why.

1. _____

2. _____

Text Reference, page 581

Discuss the differences in side effect risk of FFP compared to red blood cell transfusion.

_____

_____

_____

Text Reference, pages 581-582

Discuss platelet infusion in the neonate. Include indications, dosing and additional potential side effects.

_____

_____

_____

Text Reference, pages 582, 640

Identify two indications for whole blood transfusion in the neonate:

1. _____

2. _____

Text Reference, page 583

Discuss the use of IVIG in the neonate, including general principles, indications and potential side effects.

_____

_____

_____

Text Reference, pages 583-584

CHAPTER 43

Bleeding

Name three drugs that a mother might have taken during pregnancy that can interfere with vitamin K and synthesis of clotting factors.

1. _____

2. _____

3. _____

Text Reference, pages 586-587

PART 7 – HEMATOLOGIC DISORDERS

Give examples of the following inherited abnormalities of clotting factors.

X-linked _____

_____

Autosomal dominate _____

_____

Autosomal recessive _____

_____

Text Reference, page 587

List three potential diagnoses of the "sick" bleeding infant:

1. _____
2. _____
3. _____

Text Reference, page 589

Indicate what conditions are associated with the listed physical finding:

Petechiae _____

Large bruising _____

Abnormal retinal findings _____

Enlarged spleen _____

Text Reference, page 589

What is the purpose of the Apt test?

_____

_____

_____

Text Reference, page 590

What does an elevated D-Dimer level indicate?

_____
_____
_____

Text Reference, page 591

Discuss the following laboratory tests in relation to definition and significance of abnormal finding.

Platelet count: _____
_____

PT: _____
_____

PTT: _____
_____

Fibrinogen: _____
_____

Text Reference, page 591

Identify the five replacement therapy options for treating bleeding in the neonate:

1. _____
2. _____
3. _____
4. _____
5. _____

Text Reference, pages 592-593

Describe the treatment of DIC.

_____
_____
_____

Text Reference, page 593

PART 7 – HEMATOLOGIC DISORDERS

Describe Hemorrhagic Disease of the Newborn (HDN), including incidence, etiology, lab findings, and treatment if the infant is actively bleeding.

Text Reference, page 593-594

Describe the antenatal management of the mother who is on medication known to increase risk of HDN.

Text Reference, page 593-594

CHAPTER 44

Neonatal Thrombosis

The single greatest risk factor for arterial or venous thrombosis in the neonate is

Text Reference, page 595-596

Identify the factors that are associated with inherited prothrombotic disorders, including family history, timing and characteristics of symptoms.".

Text Reference, pages 597-598

Discuss the signs and symptoms of a catheter associated venous thrombosis.

Text Reference, page 599

Discuss the management of central catheter thrombosis.

Text Reference, pages 599-600

Name three presenting symptoms of renal vein thrombosis.

1.
2.
3.

Text Reference, page 600

Compare and contrast aortic and major arterial thrombosis.

Text Reference, pages 601-603

Discuss the advantages of low molecular weight heparin.

Text Reference, pages 606-608

_____ is the thrombolytic agent of choice for the neonate.

Text Reference, page 610

PART 7 – HEMATOLOGIC DISORDERS

CHAPTER 45

Anemia

Indicate which of the following statements about physiologic anemia of infancy are true (**T**) or false (**F**).

_____ Hemoglobin levels reach their nadir at 8 to 12 weeks of age

_____ In addition to the hematocrit level falling, the ratio of hemoglobin A to hemoglobin F also decreases

_____ After birth, erythropoietin levels rapidly increase

_____ In utero, the fetal aortic oxygen saturation is 95%

Text Reference, pages 613-614

Indicate which of the following statements or phrases about anemia of prematurity are true (**T**) or false (**F**).

_____ Vitamin E deficiency is common

_____ Iron administration will help increase the nadir of the hemoglobin levels

_____ Once the nadir is reached, iron stores stabilize

_____ RBC survival is decreased in comparison to the term infant

Text Reference, page 615

Name three obstetric causes of blood loss.

1. _____
2. _____
3. _____

Text Reference, pages 615-616

What test will determine if bleeding is fetomaternal in nature?

_____

_____

_____

Text Reference, page 616

Identify the three major causes of hemolysis:

1. _____
2. _____
3. _____

Text Reference, pages 616-617

A laboratory panel shows the following:

Increased reticulocytes, Increased bilirubin, Positive Coombs' test, Hypochromic microcytes are present.

These findings are consistent with: *check appropriate response(s)*

❏ acute hemorrhage

❏ immune hemolysis

❏ disseminated intravascular coagulation

❏ chronic fetomaternal hemorrhage

Text Reference, page 618, Table 45.3

Fill in the blanks.

The decision to transfuse must be made in consideration of the _____

and _____.

Text Reference, page 619

When should irradiated red blood cells be used for transfusion?

_____
_____
_____

Text Reference, page 622

Name at least three prophylactic measures for premature infants who are anemic.

1. _____
2. _____
3. _____

PART 7 – HEMATOLOGIC DISORDERS

Text Reference, pages 622-623

CHAPTER 46

Polycythemia

Differentiate polycythemia from hyperviscosity.

_____
_____
_____

Text Reference, page 624

Identify at least three causes of polycythemia as related to:

Placental red cell transfusion

1. _____
2. _____
3. _____

Placental insufficiency

1. _____
2. _____
3. _____

Other conditions

1. _____
2. _____
3. _____

Text Reference, pages 625-626

What is the volume of exchange in an exchange transfusion for a 3-kg infant whose hematocrit is 80% with a desired goals of hematocrit of 50%.

_____
_____
_____

Text Reference, page 628

CHAPTER 47

Neonatal Thrombocytopenia

Define thrombocytopenia.

_____

_____

_____

Text Reference, page 631

Discuss early onset thrombocytopenia.

_____

_____

_____

Text Reference, pages 631-633

The most common causes of late-onset thrombocytopenia are:

1. _____

2. _____

Text Reference, page 633-634

Describe neonatal alloimmune thrombocytopenia (NAIT).

Clinical presentation _____

_____

Pathophysiology _____

_____

Treatment (Prenatal and Postnatal) _____

_____

PART 7 – HEMATOLOGIC DISORDERS

Text Reference, pages 634-637

Describe neonatal autoimmune thrombocytopenia.

Clinical presentation _____

_____

Pathophysiology _____

_____

Treatment (Prenatal and Postnatal)_____

_____

Text Reference, pages 634-638

Discuss neonatal platelet transfusion, including optimal platelet products, how to decrease risk for CMV exposure and GVHD, and guidelines for platelet transfusion.

_____

_____

_____

_____

Text Reference, page 636, 638-640

PART 8 – INFECTIOUS DISEASES

CHAPTER 48

Viral Infections

What does the acronym TORCH stand for and why should this term be avoided?

Text Reference, page 642

Compare and contrast congenital symptomatic CMV disease with asymptomatic congenital CMV infection.

Text Reference, page 645

In suspected CMV, the specimen of greatest sensitivity can be yielded from the: *check appropriate response(s)*

❏ blood

❏ saliva

❏ urine

Text Reference, pages 646

What two drugs have been effective in the treatment of and prophylaxis against dissemination of CMV in infants?

Text Reference, page 648

PART 8 – INFECTIOUS DISEASES

What is the most common transmission route for a neonate to acquire herpes simplex virus (HSV) infection from the mother?

Text Reference, page 651

Describe the clinical symptoms of HSV infection.

Text Reference, pages 651-652

Explain why serology is of limited value in diagnosing vertically transmitted HSV in neonates.

Text Reference, page 653

Discuss management of the infant born to a woman with active genital HSV infection, including the difference in management between maternal first-episode infection and maternal recurrent infection.

Text Reference, page 654-656

What is the primary cause of pediatric AIDS?

Text Reference, page 661-662

Discuss the transmission of HIV from infected mothers to their fetuses and newborn infants, including transmission rates, the role of the placental in virus transfer and other factors affecting transmission.

Text Reference, page 661-662

Discuss the treatment of HIV in relation to Antiretroviral Therapy (ART).

Text Reference, pages 665-666

Define the following serologic findings regarding hepatitis B infection:

HBsAg _____

Anti-HBs _____

HBeAg _____

Anti-HBc _____

Text Reference, page 670

Discuss the dose and timing of the hepatitis B vaccine.

Text Reference, pages 670-671

Discuss vertical and horizontal transmission of Hepatitis C.

Text Reference, page 672

PART 8 – INFECTIOUS DISEASES

Discuss treatment of an infant who acquired perinatal varicella near the time of delivery.

Text Reference, page 675

Is the following statement true (**T**) or false (**F**)?

_____ Treatment of symptomatic enteroviral disease in the newborn is supportive only.

Text Reference, page 677

Multiple organ anomalies is most likely to occur if a fetus is exposed to rubella in: *check appropriate response*

❏ first trimester

❏ during labor and delivery

❏ third trimester

Text Reference, page 678

Discuss prevention of RSV in neonates.

Text Reference, pages 682-683

CHAPTER 49

Bacterial and Fungal Infections

Describe the symptoms and other factors regarding diagnosis of early onset sepsis.

Text Reference, pages 685-686

The recommended drug therapy for E. coli infection is _____.

Text Reference, page 687

Identify three clinical risk factors for early onset of group B streptococcal infection:

1. _____
2. _____
3. _____

Text Reference, pages 693-694

Indicate if the following statements about neonatal infection are true (**T**) or false (**F**).

_____ Term infants with late onset sepsis present with fever and/or poor feeding and lethargy.

_____ Mortality associated with P. aeruginosa sepsis is low in even low-birth-weight infants.

_____ Clindamyacin is a good alternative to amphotericin B for treatment of systemic candidiasis.

Text Reference, pages 700-712

Discuss prophylaxis against infectious conjunctivitis.

_____
_____
_____

Text Reference, page 715

Discuss the challenges associated with the diagnosis of neonatal pneumonia.

_____
_____
_____

Text Reference, pages 716-717

PART 8 – INFECTIOUS DISEASES

CHAPTER 50

Congenital Toxoplasmosis

Discuss the diagnosis of the neonate at risk for, or infected with Toxoplasmosis.

Text Reference, pages 724-725

Discuss the treatment of infected neonates.

Text Reference, page 726

CHAPTER 51

Syphilis

List the clinical signs of congenital syphilis.

Text Reference, pages 728-729

List and describe the four scenarios used by the CDC for classifying infants evaluated for congenital syphilis and describe the treatment for each scenario:

1. _____

2. _____

3. _____

4. _____

_____

Text Reference, pages 733-734

CHAPTER 52

Tuberculosis

A mother has active tuberculosis. Her neonate is asymptomatic. Management of the neonate should include: *check appropriate response(s)*

- ❏ BCG vaccine
- ❏ skin testing
- ❏ prophylactic INH

Text Reference, pages 749-750

When a mother has been diagnosed with tuberculosis, indicate when it is necessary to separate mother and baby as an infection control measure.

_____

_____

_____

Text Reference, page 750

CHAPTER 53

Lyme Disease

Discuss the treatment of mothers and the newborn with early disseminated or late disseminated Lyme disease:

Early disseminated

_____

_____

Late disseminated

_____

_____

Text Reference, pages 757-758

PART 9 – NEUROLOGIC DISORDERS

CHAPTER 54

Intracranial Hemorrhage and White Matter Injury/Periventricular Leukomalacia

What is the best predictor of outcome in a neonate with intracranial hemorrhage?

_____

_____

_____

Text Reference, page 761

Indicate which of the following statements are true (**T**) or false (**F**) about intracranial hemorrhages.

_____ The pathogenesis of subdural hemorrhage relates to rupture of veins and sinuses of the brain.

_____ When a large subdural hemorrhage is suspected, a lumbar puncture should be performed.

_____ Subarachnoid hemorrhage can be asymptomatic.

_____ Intracerebellar hemorrhage is more common in preterm neonates.

_____ The two major complications of intraventricular hemorrhage are infarction and post-hemorrhagic ventricular dilation.

_____ A factor that contributes to intraventricular hemorrhage is the fragile nature of the vessels of the germinal matrix.

Text Reference, pages 762-770

Diagnosis of subdural hemorrhage should be confirmed with:
check appropriate response(s)

❏ CT scan

❏ Ultrasound

❏ MRI

Text Reference, page 763

Discuss the grading of intraventricular hemorrhage.

_____

_____

_____

Text Reference, pages 771-772, Table 54.3

Discuss the clinical presentation and diagnosis of PVL in the neonate.

Text Reference, page 781

CHAPTER 55

Perinatal Asphyxia and Hypoxic-Ischemic Encephalopathy

Define perinatal asphyxia.

Text Reference, page 790

Differentiate the following terms by defining each. Describe clinical features where applicable.

Perinatal hypoxia _____

Perinatal ischemia _____

Perinatal asphyxia _____

Perinatal/neonatal depression _____

Neonatal encephalopathy _____

Hypoxic-ischemic brain injury _____

Text Reference, pages 790-791

PART 9 – NEUROLOGIC DISORDERS

List three factors that increase the risk of perinatal asphyxia:

1. _____
2. _____
3. _____

Text Reference, page 792

List five etiologies of hypoxia-ischemia:

1. _____
2. _____
3. _____
4. _____
5. _____

Text Reference, page 792

Compare the physiologic and biochemical alterations of brief versus prolonged asphyxia.

_____
_____
_____

Text Reference, page 793

Cellular dysfunction in asphyxia occurs as a result of:

1. _____
2. _____

Text Reference, page 793

PART 9 – NEUROLOGIC DISORDERS

Define the following terms; state the cause and sequelae of each:

Necrosis _____

_____

Apoptosis _____

_____

Reperfusion _____

_____

Text Reference, page 793

Describe the neurologic signs of HIE.

_____

_____

Text Reference, page 795

Describe and differentiate between the Sarnot Stages of HIE.

_____

_____

_____

Text Reference, pages 796-797

PART 9 – NEUROLOGIC DISORDERS

Identify the other organ systems commonly affected by asphyxia and describe specific dysfunction of each system:

1. _____

2. _____

3. _____

4. _____

5. _____

6. _____

Text Reference, pages 797-798

Describe the management of HIE in the following phases of delivery and neonatal care.

Perinatal

_____

Postnatal-Ventilation

_____

Oxygenation

_____

Temperature

_____

Perfusion and metabolic alterations

_____

Fluid management

_____

Text Reference, pages 800-802

Discuss the seizures characteristic of infants with HIE, including timing of onset and acute and long-term management.

_____

_____

_____

Text Reference, pages 802-803

Describe the management of other target organ injury.

Cardiac _____

_____

Renal _____

_____

GI _____

_____

Hematologic _____

_____

Liver _____

_____

Lung _____

_____

Text Reference, pages 803-804

List the three major inclusion criteria for therapeutic hypothermia:

1. _____

2. _____

3. _____

Text Reference, page 804

PART 9 – NEUROLOGIC DISORDERS

Specifically describe safety monitoring and management during therapeutic hypothermia.

Temperature _____

_____

Respiratory status _____

_____

Cardiovascular _____

_____

Fluid & electrolyte/renal/GI _____

_____

Infectious disease _____

_____

Neurologic status _____

_____

Pain & sedation _____

_____

Text Reference, pages 805-807

Indicate if the following statements about the prognosis of neonates with perinatal asphyxia are true (**T**) or false (**F**).

_____ There is a mortality rate of 20%.

_____ The risk of cerebral palsy is elevated 25% over the normal population.

_____ The presence of seizures increases the risk of cerebral palsy 50-70 fold.

_____ Low voltage EEG activity is an indicator of good outcomes.

Text Reference, pages 808-809

CHAPTER 56
Neonatal Seizures

Discuss the newborn brain's immaturity and how that influences clinical seizure presentation.

_____

_____

_____

Text Reference, page 812

Describe the physical characteristics of the following seizures.

A. Focal Clonic _____

B. Focal Tonic _____

C. Myoclonic _____

D. Autonomic _____

Text Reference, pages 813-815

Discuss the role of EEG in the diagnosis of seizures.

_____

_____

_____

Text Reference, page 816

Check **all** of the following statements that are **true** regarding conditions that cause neonatal seizures.

❏ In neonates with subdural hemorrhage, seizures may be associated with cerebral contusion

❏ Neonates with hypoglycemia are at risk for seizures

❏ Infections may lead to seizures

❏ Seizures are not a result of cerebral dysgenesis

❏ Infants with pyridoxine dependency often outgrow this condition around one year of age

Text Reference, pages 819-822

PART 9 – NEUROLOGIC DISORDERS

Identify three drug therapies for neonatal seizures:

1. _____
2. _____
3. _____

Text Reference, pages 825-827

Check **all** of the following statements that are **true** in terms of prognosis for neonates with seizures.

❑ Improved outcomes occur with increasing gestational age.

❑ EEGs are not useful in determining prognosis.

❑ Mortality rates are less than 20%.

❑ Underlying etiology is the most important factor affecting outcomes.

❑ Mortality and morbidity rates have both decreased in recent years.

Text Reference, page 827

CHAPTER 57

Neural Tube Defects

List the two types of neural tube defects; identify and describe three examples each.

1. _____
   _____
   _____

2. _____
   _____
   _____

Text Reference, pages 829-830

Fill in the blanks.

The overall frequency of neural tube defects is _____.

Etiologies for both primary and secondary neural tube defects are _____.

As a preventive measure it is recommended that pregnant women take _____ daily.

Text Reference, page 830-831

Discuss the possible advantages of *in utero* repair in patients with myelomeningocele. Identify the complication risks.

Text Reference, page 836

Discuss the preoperative management of myleomeningocele, including care of the defect, prevention of infection, urinary catheterization, latex allergy and management of hydrocephalus."

Text Reference, page 837-838

An increased risk of cognitive delay in neonates with neural tube defects is associated with:

1.
2.
3.
4.
5.

Text Reference, page 841

PART 10 – BONE CONDITIONS

CHAPTER 58

Orthopedic Problems

Fill in the blanks.

Torticollis is caused by a shortening of the _____ muscle.

Text Reference, page 845

Treatment for torticollis involves: **check appropriate response(s)**

❏ immediate surgery

❏ immobilization of the head

❏ passive stretching exercises

Text Reference, page 846

List the three types of hip dislocation:

1. _____
2. _____
3. _____

Text Reference, page 849

Indicate if the following statements about classic dislocation of the hip are true (**T**) or false (**F**).

_____ It is diagnosed by a positive Ortolani sign

_____ Asymmetry of the pelvis is common

_____ The hip dislocates on adduction

_____ X-rays confirm diagnosis

_____ Ultrasound is used to monitor the condition

_____ It affects more females than males

Text Reference, pages 847-849

Match the statement with the following deformities of the feet. **More than one answer may apply**.

a. Nonstructural metatarsus adductus

b. Calcaneovalgus deformities

c. Congenital clubfoot

d. Structural metatarus adductus

_____ Appearance doesn't always correlate with severity of the condition

_____ It is caused by in utero positioning

_____ A short leg cast may be necessary

_____ It has a multifactorial etiology

_____ Treatment is not needed

_____ It is associated with oligohydramnios

Text Reference, pages 850-851

CHAPTER 59

Osteopenia (Metabolic Bone Disease) of Prematurity

What are the principal causes of metabolic bone disease of prematurity?

_____

_____

_____

Text Reference, page 853

Differentiate between osteopenia and rickets.

_____

_____

_____

Text Reference, page 854

Describe the clinical sign of metabolic bone disease including x-ray findings.

_____

_____

_____

Text Reference, pages 854-855

PART 10 – BONE CONDITIONS

The laboratory finding that is considered the earliest indicator of osteopenia is:

Text Reference, page 855

Identify preventive strategies for metabolic bone disease.

Text Reference, pages 856-857

PART 11 – METABOLISM

CHAPTER 60

Inborn Errors of Metabolism (IEM)

List the clinical groups in which neonates with IEM present:

1. _____
2. _____
3. _____
4. _____

Text Reference, page 859

Check **all** of the following statements that are **true** about inborn errors of metabolism.

- ❏ Many of the diseases present with feeding problems
- ❏ Elevated direct and indirect bilirubin occurs with galactosemia
- ❏ The presence of ketonuria rules out metabolic defects

Text Reference, pages 859, 862, 866-867

Describe the first line laboratory studies that should be initiated for neonates suspected of having an inborn error of metabolism.

_____
_____
_____

Text Reference, pages 864-866, Table 60.7

In urea cycle disorders, laboratory findings that are consistent with the disease are:

1. _____
2. _____
3. _____

Text Reference, pages 874-876

PART 11 – METABOLISM

Discuss hypoglycemia with and without ketosis.

_____

_____

_____

Text Reference, page 879, Figure 60.5

List the IEM associated with seizures:

1. _____
2. _____
3. _____
4. _____
5. _____
6. _____

Text Reference, pages 882-884

Describe the physical symptoms of galactosemia.

_____

_____

_____

Text Reference, page 887

PART 12 – ENDOCRINOLOGY

CHAPTER 61

Thyroid Disorders

Discuss associated fetal/neonatal outcomes to maternal hypothyroidism.

_____

_____

_____

Text Reference, page 895

Describe normal thyroid physiology in the newborn period.

_____

_____

_____

Text Reference, pages 896-897

Congenital hypothyroidism is one of the _____ common preventable causes of _____ _____.

Text Reference, page 897

Compare and contrast the clinical symptoms of neonatal hyperthyroidism and congenital hypothyroidism.

_____

_____

_____

Text Reference, pages 897-908

Discuss the cause of transient congenital hypothyroidism.

_____

_____

_____

Text Reference, pages 900-902

PART 12 – ENDOCRINOLOGY

Discuss maternal thyroid medications and breast feeding.

_____
_____
_____

Text Reference, page 908

CHAPTER 62

Neonatal Effects of Maternal Diabetes

There is an increased risk of intrauterine growth restriction in pregnancies where the diabetic woman also has: *check appropriate response(s)*

- ❏ polyhydramnios
- ❏ high first trimester glucose levels
- ❏ vascular disease

Text Reference, page 913

Discuss the following effects of maternal DM on the neonate:

Mortality _____
_____

Prematurity _____
_____

Large for gestational age _____
_____

Respiratory distress _____
_____

Hypoglycemia _____
_____

Hypocalcemia _____
_____

Hypomagnesemia _____
_____

Discuss the following effects of maternal DM on the neonate:

Hyperbilirubinemia _____
_____

Polycythemia/RVT _____
_____

Small left colon_____
_____

Hypertrophic cardiomyopathy _____
_____

Poor feeding _____
_____

Text Reference, page 916-919

Identify two complications that specifically affect LGA infants of diabetic mothers:

1._____
2._____

Text Reference, page 917

Describe the post-delivery management of IDMs according to presenting symptoms and continued evaluation.

asymptomatic with normal blood glucose

_____
_____
_____

symptomatic with low blood glucose after enteral feedings

_____
_____
_____

Text Reference, pages 920-921

PART 12 – ENDOCRINOLOGY

List four long-term effects in infants of diabetic mothers:

1. _____
2. _____
3. _____
4. _____

Text Reference, pages 920-922

CHAPTER 63

Disorders of Sex Development

Aside from parental concerns regarding sex assignment, why should the evaluation of a newborn with suspected disorder of sex development (DSD) **not** be delayed?

_____

_____

Text Reference, page 923

Identify key factors in the patient history of a baby with DSD that should be explored:

1. _____
2. _____
3. _____
4. _____
5. _____

Text Reference, pages 927

Discuss the three key components in the physical assessment of a neonate with suspected DSD.

1. _____
2. _____
3. _____

Text Reference, pages 927-928

Discuss the diagnostic tests utilized in the evaluation for DSD.

Text Reference, pages 929-932

Discuss the diagnosis and management of congenital adrenal hyperplasia (CAH).

Text Reference, pages 934-937

Sex assignment in the case of ambiguous genitalia remains controversial. Key considerations include:
check appropriate response(s)

- ❏ Anatomy and functional endocrinology
- ❏ Chromosomal analysis
- ❏ Parents' preference
- ❏ Ability to preserve fertility

Text Reference, pages 940-941

PART 13 – SURGERY

CHAPTER 64

Surgical Emergencies in the Newborn

Discuss the significance of the following perinatal findings related to potential surgical conditions in the neonate.

Polyhydramnios _____

_____

Oligohydramnios _____

_____

Meconium peritonitis _____

_____

Fetal ascites _____

_____

Dystocia _____

_____

Text Reference, pages 942-943

Identify neonatal disorders that may be associated with each of the following symptoms:

Respiratory distress _____

_____

Scaphoid abdomen _____

_____

Excessive mucous and salivation _____

_____

Pneumoperitoneum _____

_____

Bilious emesis _____

_____

Nonbilious emesis _____

_____

Failure to pass meconium _____

_____

Failure to develop transitional stools _____

Hematochezia _____

Abdominal masses _____

Text Reference, pages 944-947

Describe esophageal atresia and its association with tracheoesophoageal fistula.

_____

Text Reference, pages 947-948

Describe congenital diaphragmatic hernia in relation to symptoms, diagnosis, and airway maintenance.

_____

Text Reference, pages 949-950

Describe the following neonatal anomalies and identify respiratory symptoms specific to each.

Congenital lobar emphysema _____

Choanal atresia _____

Pierre Robin syndrome _____

Text Reference, pages 951-952

What is the most critical lesion to rule out in the neonate with suspected intestinal obstruction?

_____

Text Reference, page 952

PART 13 – SURGERY

List examples of the following types of intestinal obstruction:

Congenital mechanical obstruction _____

_____

Acquired mechanical obstruction _____

_____

Functional intestinal obstruction _____

_____

Text Reference, page 953

Describe duodenal atresia in relation to associated malformation, symptoms, and diagnostic criteria.

_____

_____

_____

Text Reference, pages 953-954

Describe meconium ileus including symptoms, associated disorders, and medical management.

_____

_____

_____

Text Reference, pages 954-955

Discuss imperforate anus including associated anomalies, characteristics, and treatment of each.

_____

_____

_____

Text Reference, page 955

What are the symptoms of malrotation of the bowel? How is the diagnosis made and why is intestinal obstruction caused by malrotation a surgical emergency?

___

Text Reference, page 955

Define and give characteristics of clinical presentation of the following defects:

Hirschsprung's disease ___

Meconium or mucous plug syndrome ___

Annular pancreas ___

Text Reference, pages 956-957

Compare and contrast omphalocele and gastroschisis.

___

Text Reference, pages 957-958

Briefly describe the following renal disorders, including symptoms, pre-operative management (if applicable), and treatment.

Genitourinary abnormalities ___

Renal vein thrombosis ___

Exstrophy of the bladder ___

Text Reference, pages 958-959

PART 13 – SURGERY

What are the two most common malignant tumors in the newborn?

___

Text Reference, page 960

What are the factors for determining whether repair of inguinal hernia should occur before discharge or at a later date?

___

Text Reference, pages 960-961

Describe the differential diagnosis of the neonate with scrotal swelling.

___

Text Reference, pages 961-962

Briefly describe the use of the following diagnostic tests:

Contrast enema ___

Ultrasound ___

CT ___

Immunoreactive trypsin ___

Text Reference, pages 962-963

Describe preoperative management of the infant with the following presenting symptom(s):

Vomiting without distension _____

_____

Nonbilious vomiting with distension _____

_____

Bilious vomiting with distension _____

_____

Masses _____

_____

Text Reference, pages 963-965

PART 14 – DERMATOLOGY

CHAPTER 65

Skin Care

Discuss the following neonatal skin care practices appropriate to eliminating or minimizing skin injury.

Bathing _____

_____

Use of adhesives _____

_____

Cord care _____

_____

Humidity _____

_____

Circumcision care _____

_____

Disinfectants _____

_____

Emollients _____

_____

Text Reference, pages 968-970

Discuss the aspects of wound care in relation to:

Common causes of neonatal wounds _____

Identification of stages of wound healing _____

Essential elements of wound management _____

Use of wound dressings and products _____

Text Reference, pages 971-972

Discuss the following aspects of extravasation prevention and management.

Prevention _____

_____

Treatment _____

_____

Administration of antidotes _____

Text Reference, pages 972-973

Describe the following common transient cutaneous lesions of:

Milia _____

Sebaceous gland hyperplasia _____

Erythemia toxicum _____

Incontinence associated diaper dermatitis _____

Text Reference, pages 973-974

Describe abnormalities of pigmentation and the significance, if any, to underlying disease.

_____

_____

_____

Text Reference, pages 974-975

List developmental abnormalities of the skin and the significance of each:

_____

_____

_____

Text Reference, pages 975-976

What skin conditions are classified as scaling skin disorders?

_____

_____

_____

Text Reference, page 976

What skin disorders are classified as vesicobullous eruptions?

_____

_____

Text Reference, pages 976

PART 15 – VASCULAR ANOMALIES

CHAPTER 66

Vascular Anomalies

Describe infantile hemangioma.

Presenting signs & symptoms _____

_____

Usual management _____

_____

Possible complications _____

_____

Usual progression of lesion _____

_____

Management of more significant or complicated lesions _____

_____

Text Reference, pages 978-982

Describe the difference between infantile hemangioma and congenital hemangioma.

_____

_____

Text Reference, pages 978-982

Identify the two forms of congenital hemangioma and the management of each:

1. _____

_____

2. _____

_____

Text Reference, page 982

PART 15 – VASCULAR ANOMALIES

Define the following vascular malformations and recommended treatments:

Capillary malformations _____
_____

Lymphatic malformations _____
_____

Venous malformations _____
_____

Arteriovenous malformations _____
_____

Text Reference, pages 983-984

PART 16 – AUDITORY AND OPTHALMOLOGIC DISORDERS

CHAPTER 67

Retinopathy of Prematurity (ROP)

Describe retinopathy of prematurity (ROP), including pathogenesis, possible mechanisms of injury, and risk factors.

_____
_____
_____

Identify appropriate screening criteria for ROP.

_____
_____
_____

Text Reference, pages 986-987

Describe the classification of ROP based on the following components:

Location _____
_____

Severity _____
_____

Plus disease _____
_____

Extent _____

Text Reference, page 988

Define the following terms:

Agressive posterior ROP _____
_____

Threshold ROP _____
_____

Prethreshold ROP - Type 1 _____
_____

Prethreshold ROP - Type 2 _____

Text Reference, pages 988-990

Complete the following statements:

Current recommendations are to consider treatment for the eyes with:

_____

Close observation is recommended for:

_____

Text Reference, pages 990

Discuss both short- and long-term prognosis for infants with ROP based on location of disease, severity of stage, circumferential involvement, presence of plus disease and how fast the disease progresses.

_____

_____

_____

_____

Text Reference, pages 990-991

Discuss the following treatment modalities for ROP.

Anti-VEGF therapy _____

_____

Cryotherapy _____

_____

Laser therapy _____

_____

Retinal reattachment _____

_____

Text Reference, pages 991-992

PART 16 – AUDITORY AND OPTHALMOLOGIC DISORDERS

CHAPTER 68

Hearing Loss in Neonatal Intensive Care Unit Graduates

Differentiate between sensorineural and conductive hearing loss.

_____

_____

_____

Text Reference, page 993

What percentage of congenital hearing loss is thought to be of:

   Genetic origin: _____

   Nongenetic origin: _____

What is the most common cause of nonhereditary sensorineural hearing loss?

_____

Text Reference, page 994

List the risk factors for hearing loss in NICU graduates.

_____

_____

_____

Text Reference, page 995

Compare these hearing screening tests.

ABR _____

_____

_____

EOAE _____

_____

_____

Text Reference, page 996

The prognosis for hearing loss is dependent on _____ ,

_____ , as well as

. _____

Text Reference, page 998

PART 17 – COMMON NEONATAL PROCEDURES

CHAPTER 69

Common Neonatal Procedures

Describe the general principles when performing procedures on neonates.

_____
_____
_____

Text Reference, pages 1000-1002

Describe correct procedure for capillary blood sampling, including applicable blood studies, preparation of site, equipment used, and appropriate sites for heel sticks.

_____
_____
_____

Text Reference, page 1002

Discuss the following in relation to lumbar puncture procedure in neonates.

    Technique: _____

    Significance of:

        RBC count: _____

        WBC count: _____

        Glucose/protein levels: _____

Text Reference, pages 1003-1006

Describe the appropriate technique for neonatal endotracheal intubation.

_____
_____
_____

Text Reference, pages 1006-1008

Describe the correct method for insertion/removal of umbilical artery catheters.

Text Reference, pages 1009-1013

Describe problems and complications that may occur with umbilical artery catheterization.

Text Reference, pages 1013-1014

What are the indications, advantages, and risks for the following:

Percutaneous radial artery catheterization: _____

Percutaneous central venous catheterization: _____

Abdominal paracentesis: _____

Text Reference, pages 1017-1019

PART 18 – PAIN AND STRESS CONTROL

CHAPTER 70

Preventing and Treating Pain and Stress Among Infants in the Intensive Care Unit

Regarding fetal and neonatal responses to pain, complete the following sentences:

There is considerable maturation of peripheral, spinal, and supraspinal neurologic pathways for response to painful stimuli by late in the _____ trimester.

By _____ weeks gestation, cutaneous sensory nerve terminals are present in all body areas.

Text Reference, pages 1022-1023

Infants exhibit predictable pain response patterns with respect to:

1. _____
2. _____
3. _____
4. _____

Text Reference, pages 1022-1023

Describe neonatal medical and developmental outcomes specific to the following.

Medical and surgical outcomes _____

Neurodevelopmental outcomes _____

Text Reference, pages 1023-1024

Identify the AAP's Principles of Prevention and Management of Neonatal Pain and Stress.

1. _____
2. _____
3. _____
4. _____

5. _____

6. _____

7. _____

Text Reference, page 1024

Describe pain prevention and treatment relative to:

Environmental and behavioral approaches _____

Physiological interventions _____

Text Reference, pages 1028, 1031-1032

What are components of the Neonatal Pain Assessment Tools?

_____

Text Reference, pages 1026-1027

Match the drugs that should be administered for the procedures being performed on neonates

A. Sucrose
B. Short acting opioid
C. Lidocaine
D. Acetaminophen
E. EMLA

_____ Lumbar puncture
_____ IV insertion
_____ Chest tube insertion
_____ Peripheral arterial catheter placement
_____ Eye Exam

_____ Circumcision
_____ Immunization injection
_____ Heel stick blood draw
_____ Intubation
_____ PICC

Text Reference, pages 1029-1031, 1035

PRACTICE TEST

1) A nuchal translucency is done at 12 weeks that shows an increased nuchal thickening. Additional testing may include
   A. biophysical profile
   B. fetal echocardiogram
   C. percutaneous umbilical blood sampling

2) The presence of maternal hyperglycemia places the neonate at risk for
   A. hypercalcemia
   B. hyperglycemia
   C. hyperinsulinemia

3) A mother is admitted to the birthing center due to declining renal function and severe headache with visual changes. She is carrying 24 week twins and has been on bed rest for the past 8 weeks. After 48 hours the mother's headache and visual changes persist. The clinician can expect
   A. antihypertensive therapy to be initiated
   B. induction of labor is likely
   C. the mother's diet will be modified to restrict salt intake

4) A neonate born to a mother given Demerol three hours prior to delivery is apneic and cyanotic with heart rate of 74 at one hour after birth. The initial intervention should be
   A. administration of naloxone 0.1mg/kg
   B. bag and mask ventilation
   C. placement of endotracheal tube

5) What size endotracheal tube should be available to resuscitate a 36 week 2500g newborn?
   A. 2.5 mm
   B. 3.0 mm
   C. 3.5 mm

6) Hydrops Fetalis involves extracellular fluid in
   A. 2 or more body compartments
   B. the abdomen
   C. the lungs and heart

7) Following a traumatic delivery, a neonate's arm falls motionless along the side of the body and is rotated inwards. Extension of the forearm is present and grasp reflex is intact. This infant likely has
   A. Erb's Palsy
   B. Klumpke Palsy
   C. Total Brachial Plexus Injury

8) To confirm or supplement obstetric dating for infants at 20-24 weeks gestation, the following should be used
   A. Ballard Newborn Maturity Rating
   B. Dubowitz Clinical Assessment of Gestational Age
   C. Lubchenco Clinical Estimation of Gestational Age

9) A neonate born at 36 weeks gestation had Apgar scores of 8 and 8 and appears to be physiologically stable. The nurse notes that the infant has hiccups, frequent yawns and occasionally sneezes. These are signs of
   A. autonomic stress
   B. normal first period of reactivity
   C. self-regulation

10) When following safe sleep guidelines, a baby sleeps on
    A. his/her side
    B. prone
    C. supine

11) Teratogenic agents are most likely to cause birth defects when the fetus is exposed during the
    A. 4th-7th weeks of gestation
    B. 8th-12th weeks of gestation
    C. 13th-17th weeks gestation

12) What are the characteristics of a dizygotic pregnancy?
    A. 1 placenta and 1 amniotic sac
    B. 1 placenta and 2 amniotic sacs
    C. 2 placentas, 2 chorions and 2 amniotic sacs

13) The AAP recommends that opioid exposed infants remain in the hospital for a minimum of
    A. 48 hours
    B. 72 hours
    C. 96 hours

14) Potential outcomes of neonates who were exposed to cocaine in utero include

    A. drug withdrawal
    B. neurobehavior abnormalities
    C. physical anomalies

15) A woman on methadone wants to breastfeed. She should be advised that

    A. methadone is incompatible with breastfeeding
    B. she may as long as she remains in a substance abuse treatment program
    C. the baby needs to be supplemented with formula

16) An 800g 26 week infant has a mean blood pressure of 20mm Hg at 12 hours of life. The most likely cause of this infant's hypotension is

    A. altered vasoreactivity
    B. fetal magnesium exposure
    C. hypovolemia

17) When repositioning infants it is important to provide

    A. extension of extremities
    B. limitation of movement
    C. midline alignment

18) A neutral thermal environment is the environmental temperature in which body temperature is maintained and

    A. energy expenditure is minimized
    B. metabolic rate is maximized
    C. skin and core temperature gradient is small

19) Risk of blindness due to ROP in the ELBW population is

    A. < 1%
    B. 1-2%
    C. > 2%

20) After an initial resuscitation, poor perfusion continues, pulses are thready, and the neonate appears in shock. Dopamine is administered as a continuous IV infusion. The transport nurse should recognize that

    A. beneficial effects are dependent on adequate blood volume
    B. increased blood pressure can be expected at low doses
    C. the serum half-life is 1-2 minutes

21) When there is a surviving multiple (twin, triplet, etc.) the team should acknowledge

    A. how this will ease the pain and suffering of the family
    B. the difficulty this will present during the grieving process
    C. the surviving infant may have difficulty bonding with parents

22) When comparing the same volume of mature human milk and premature human milk, the mature milk has less

    A. carbohydrates
    B. fat
    C. protein

23) A two week old premature infant exhibits fussiness, gagging and poor feeding behavior. Gastroesophageal reflux (GER) is the suspected diagnosis. The nurse should know that

    A. 25% of GER patients require prolonged medical management
    B. physiologic GER resolves in most infants by 8-10 months
    C. symptoms usually respond to alterations in feeding regimen

24) A breastfeeding mother develops redness on her right breast accompanied by fever, chills and headache. In addition to antibiotic therapy, an appropriate intervention would be

    A. cold compresses to the affected breast
    B. continue breastfeeding to empty affected breast
    C. discontinue breast feeding until the symptoms subside

25) A breastfeeding baby should return to birth weight by how many days of life?

    A. 8-9
    B. 12-14
    C. 15-17

26) Low urinary chloride can be caused by

    A. diuretic therapy
    B. soy formula
    C. vomiting

PRACTICE TEST

27) In the term infant the percentage of weight loss in the first 5 to 6 days is
    A. 1-2%
    B. 3-5%
    C. 6-8%

28) An extremely premature neonate is hyperglycemic with a serum glucose of 250mg/dL. The provider orders a one-time does of insulin. The correct dose is
    A. 0.05 to 0.1 units/kg
    B. 0.11 to 0.2 units/kg
    C. 0.21 to 0.25 units/kg

29) Calcium levels usually decline for the first 24-48 hours after birth. The nadir of neonatal calcium for a healthy term infant is
    A. 6.5 to 7.4mg/dL
    B. 7.5 to 8.4mg/dL
    C. 8.5 to 9.4mg/dL

30) Regarding neonatal hypercalcemia, the upper limit of normal for serum total calcium is
    A. 7 mg/dL
    B. 11 mg/dL
    C. 13 mg/dL

31) Which of the following is a true statement regarding neonatal hyperbilirubinemia?
    A. Conjugated bilirubin is reabsorbed in the intestine
    B. In VLBW infants, albumin has an increased affinity for bilirubin
    C. Newborn infants produce more bilirubin per day than adults

32) Bronze baby syndrome is caused by phototherapy in a baby with which of the following conditions?
    A. Direct hyperbilirubinemia
    B. Glucose-6-phosphate dehydrogenase (G6PD
    C. Isoimmune hemolytic disease

33) The primary cause of most cholestasis or conjugated hyperbilirubinemia in the NICU is
    A. congenital obstructive bile duct disease
    B. prolonged exposure to parenteral nutrition
    C. viral or bacterial sepsis

34) The x-ray of a neonate with suspected necrotizing enterocolitis shows pneumoperitoneum. This finding is consistent with
    A. air in the portal venous system
    B. diffuse gaseous intestinal distention
    C. intestinal perforation

35) NEC in term infants most commonly affects the
    A. colon
    B. rectum
    C. small intestine

36) Aminoglycosides are a factor in which renal disease category?
    A. Intrinsic
    B. Obstructive
    C. Prerenal

37) Which of the following statements regarding Continuous Positive Airway Pressure (CPAP) is true?
    A. can be administered by nasal prongs, nasopharyngeal tube or endotracheal tube
    B. decreases the risk of pneumothorax
    C. prevents alveolar and airway collapse

38) When considering noninvasive capnography, the clinician should know that
    A. end-tidal measurements are accurate in infants with parenchymal lung disease
    B. mainstream devices increase mechanical dead space
    C. side-stream systems require high-flow oxygen rates via nasal cannula

39) Administration of supplemental oxygen is most effective in treatment for hypoxemia resulting from
    A. diffusion impairment
    B. hypoventilation
    C. shunt

40) Most apnea spells in the preterm infant are
    A. central
    B. mixed
    C. obstructive

41) Apnea of prematurity
    A. is closely associated with periodic breathing
    B. may be increased by a cool environment
    C. will most likely present in the first week of life

42) Which condition increases the neonate's risk for transient tachypnea of the newborn (TTN)?
    A. Cesarean birth
    B. Rupture of membranes >12 hours
    C. Unmedicated labor

43) By 24 weeks gestation, which of the following is adequately developed to provide gas exchange in the ELBW newborn?
    A. Basic lung structure
    B. Surfactant stores
    C. The number of alveolar type II cells

44) The key principle in the management of respiratory distress syndrome is to
    A. establish and maintain functional residual capacity
    B. increase surface tension in delicate airways
    C. minimize barotrauma and further lung injury

45) The chest x-ray appearance of infants in early stages of bronchopulmonary dysplasia is
    A. diffuse haziness and increased density
    B. multifocal ground glass opacities and areas of consolidation
    C. regions of opacification and hyperlucency

46) What type of mechanical ventilation appears to reduce the incidence of bronchopulmonary dysplasia and pulmonary air leak?
    A. High frequency oscillatory ventilation
    B. Pressure limited ventilation
    C. Volume targeted ventilation

47) When meconium aspiration syndrome is suspected, x-ray findings that would be consistent with this diagnosis are
    A. hyperinflation
    B. peripherial air bronchograms
    C. reticulogranular pattern

48) Approximately how many deliveries are complicated by meconium stained amniotic fluid?
    A. 5-10%
    B. 10-15%
    C. 15-20%

49) The most commonly associated diagnosis with persistent pulmonary hypertension of the newborn is
    A. meconium aspiration syndrome
    B. pneumonia of bacterial origin
    C. severe fetal hypoxemia

50) In an effort to decrease the hemodynamic shunt in infants with persistent pulmonary hypertension of the newborn, the treatment goal is to maintain the systemic blood pressure
    A. equal to pulmonary vascular resistance
    B. higher than pulmonary vascular resistance
    C. lower than pulmonary vascular resistance

51) The underlying pathogenesis of pulmonary hemorrhage remains unclear. Supportive treatment is recommended, including
    A. administration of packed red blood cells
    B. avoiding use of elevated peak inspiratory pressure greater than 4cm
    C. frequent suctioning to keep airway clear

52) The precise pathophysiology underlying pulmonary hemorrhage remains uncertain. However, a predisposing condition that may initiate hemorrhage in the neonatal lung is
    A. acute right ventricular failure
    B. an alteration in the integrity of the alveolar epithelial-endothelial barrier
    C. thrombocytopenia and coagulation disorder

53) A chest x-ray reveals a hypertranslucent hemothorax on an asymptomatic full-term newborn 6 hours post-Caesarean delivery. The infant required positive-pressure ventilation in the delivery room. What is the appropriate management?
    A. Close observation
    B. Oxygen therapy for 24-48 hours
    C. Thoracentesis with "butterfly" needle or IV catheter

PRACTICE TEST

54) At 36 hours of age a 28 week gestation premature infant is intubated and placed on a ventilator. The infant's condition gradually deteriorates with heart rate < 100bpm and blood pressure of 30/16. ABG results are pH-7.25, PaO_2-32, $PaCO_2$-58. Chest x-ray appearance is linear radiolucencies radiating from the lung helium. What is the likely diagnosis?
   A. Pneumopericardium
   B. Pneumothorax
   C. Pulmonary interstitial emphysema

55) During ECMO poor venous return to the circuit causes the pump to shut down in order to prevent
   A. air entrapment
   B. clotting in the circuit
   C. volume overload

56) A full term neonate on ECMO day 5 has fluid overload. What is the expected treatment while on ECMO?
   A. Continuous renal replacement therapy
   B. Hemodialysis
   C. Hemofiltration

57) Which inotrope's effect on myocardial contractility is dependent on myocardial norepinephrine stores?
   A. Dobutamine
   B. Dopamine
   C. Epinephrine

58) A newborn is diagnosed with cyanotic heart disease. Which of the following is an example of this type of congenital heart defect?
   A. Coarctation of the aorta
   B. Ebstein's anomaly
   C. Ventricular septal defect

59) What percentage of congenital heart defects are considered critical congenital heart disease requiring intervention in the first year of life?
   A. 20
   B. 25
   C. 30

60) 30 minutes after initiation of PGE_1 on an infant with suspected cardiac anomaly, the patient's condition worsens. Which category of lesions would the clinician be most concerned with?
   A. Left atrial hypertension
   B. Left ventricle hypertension
   C. Right ventricle hypertension

61) What percentage of infants with complete atrioventricular canal have Trisomy 21?
   A. 60%
   B. 70%
   C. 80%

62) A 3500g term infant male is born to a 35 y/o G1P0 and noted to have persistent platelet counts less than 50,000. A diagnosis of neonatal alloimmune thrombocytopenia is made. Which would be an appropriate treatment for this infant?
   A. Fresh frozen plasma
   B. Intravenous immunoglobulin
   C. Platelets

63) The occurrence of newborn hemorrhagic disease in infants who do not receive vitamin K is one out of every
   A. 200-400 infants
   B. 500-700 infants
   C. 800-1000 infants

64) Which diagnostic test should be performed in all cases of suspected aortic thrombosis?
   A. Contrast study
   B. Echocardiogram
   C. Ultrasound

65) A preterm infant born at 24 weeks gestation has persistent respiratory failure and pale color despite resuscitation. The initial hematocrit is 15. What test would you consider requesting to determine if fetomaternal bleeding occurred?
   A. Apt test
   B. D-dimer assay
   C. Kleihauer-Betke stain

66) Which condition is most associated with polycythemia?
    A. Beckwith-Weideman Syndrome
    B. Turner Syndrome
    C. Von-Willebrand Syndrome

67) The most frequent cause of thrombocytopenia in an asymptomatic neonate in the first 72 hours of life is
    A. bacterial infection
    B. necrotizing enterocolitis (NEC)
    C. placental insufficiency

68) A 38-week gestation neonate is born to a HIV positive mother who has not received prenatal care. The clinician should be aware that the rate of HIV transmission from untreated infected mothers to their newborns is estimated to be between
    A. 15-40%
    B. 50-75%
    C. 80-90%

69) The most common presenting symptom of early onset sepsis is
    A. hypoglycemia
    B. respiratory distress
    C. temperature instability

70) Recent evidence reveals the drug of choice to prevent Candida infection in VLBW infants is
    A. amphotericin B
    B. fluconazole
    C. nystatin

71) Congenital toxoplasmosis is most often secondary to
    A. acute maternal infection during pregnancy
    B. reactivation of previous infection in immunocompromised mother
    C. women infected within three months of conception

72) Which of the following descriptions describes the clinical presentation of most neonates affected by congenital syphilis?
    A. Asymptomatic
    B. Generalized rash
    C. Premature

73) If the mother of a newborn has a positive TB test and a normal chest x-ray, which of the following describes appropriate management of her infant?
    A. Delay discharge until other family members are tested for TB. Mother may begin breastfeeding infant.
    B. Do not delay discharge, but test family members for TB. Mother may breastfeed.
    C. Do not delay discharge, but test family members for TB. Mother should not breastfeed because of risk of transmission of TB to infant.

74) Early case reports and case studies have documented that transplacental transmission of B. burgborferi is possible. Women who are seropositive for B. burgborferi with their first prenatal visit and at the time of delivery are more likely to have a newborn with:
    A. congenital infection
    B. low birth weight
    C. no adverse neonatal outcome

75) A neonate with a moderate subarachnoid hemorrhage is being discharged. The parents are concerned about the infant's potential problems. The clinician should advise that
    A. cerebral palsy is a rare occurrence
    B. chronic meningitis is likely
    C. hydrocephalus may occur

76) According to the Volpe grading system, an intraventricular hemorrhage that occupies 10-50% of ventricular area on parasagittal view would be a
    A. Grade I
    B. Grade II
    C. Grade III

77) Which of the following statements correctly describes seizures caused by hypoxic-ischemic encephalopathy?
    A. Seizures are often subclinical and difficult to monitor.
    B. Seizures can usually be controlled by anticonvulsant medications.
    C. Seizures generally start within six hours of birth and resolve over a few weeks.

PRACTICE TEST

78) Simultaneous fast rhythmic contractions of extremities with slower relaxation phase describes what type of neonatal seizure?
    A. Focal clonic
    B. Focal tonic
    C. Myoclonic

79) In the neonatal brain, clinical seizures are reflective of
    A. diminished connectivity of neurons
    B. excessive hyperpolarization of neurons
    C. excitatory neurotransmitters

80) What is the most common way a developmental dislocation of the hip is diagnosed in a newborn?
    A. Physical examination
    B. Ultrasound
    C. X-Ray

81) An indication of congenital anomaly of the femur is
    A. a dimple on the buttocks
    B. asymmetry of thigh folds
    C. limitation of hip abduction

82) What lab screening provides the earliest indication of osteopenia of prematurity?
    A. Serum alkaline phosphatase level
    B. Serum calcium level
    C. Serum phosphorus level

83) Glycogen Storage Disease Type II (Pompe Disease) is associated with which of the following in the neonate?
    A. Cardiomyopathy
    B. Liver dysfunction
    C. Neurologic disease

84) Pyruvate dehydrogenase deficiency (PDH) is usually inherited by which pattern of inheritance?
    A. Autosomal dominate
    B. Autosomal recessive
    C. X-linked

85) A neonate has a low T4 and elevated TSH. The appropriate next step would be
    A. begin thyroid hormone replacement therapy
    B. monitor the infant for lethargy, hypotonia and feeding difficulties
    C. recheck T4 and TSH levels at two months of age

86) Small left colon syndrome can be treated with
    A. bowel training
    B. colon resection
    C. enemas

87) Fetal and neonatal mortality is caused by stillbirths, birth asphyxia, hypoxic ischemic encephalopathy and intra-amniotic infections is most closely associated with which type of maternal diabetes?
    A. Gestational
    B. Type 1
    C. Type 2

88) Rapid evaluation of an infant with suspected congenital adrenal hyperplasia is critical to prevent
    A. cardiac arrhythmia
    B. renal failure
    C. severe dehydration

89) During a morning assessment of a 26 week gestation neonate who is now DOL #15 the clinician observes the following: distended tense abdomen, BP 30/15, poor perfusion and bloody stools. Which condition should be suspected?
    A. Midgut volvulus
    B. Necrotizing enterocolitis
    C. Sepsis with ileus

90) A term neonate who has just come off mechanical ventilation and begun enteric feedings has developed abdominal distention and bile stained emesis. An x-ray depicts distended bowel that may be granular in appearance or may show tiny bubbles. These clinical and x-ray findings are consistent with
    A. malrotation with volvulus
    B. meconium ileus
    C. necrotizing enterocolitis

91) An infant admitted for suspected sepsis develops a red, excoriated and bleeding diaper rash, with scattered yellow pustules. In addition to keeping the area dry and clean, additional intervention should include application of
    A. antibiotic ointment
    B. antifungal ointment
    C. barrier cream

92) The adhesive removal method that reduces the risk of epidermal stripping in the premature infant is the use of
    A. Adhesive removers
    B. Alcohol pads
    C. Warm sterile water

93) An anomaly that typically arises postnatally and demonstrates endothelial proliferation is a vascular
    A. Deformity
    B. Malformation
    C. Tumor

94) After the initial ophthalmologic exam for a neonate in the NICU that revealed immature retina, when should the neonate be rescreened?
    A. One week
    B. Two weeks
    C. Three weeks

95) A 30 week gestation neonate was screened for Retinopathy of Prematurity. The findings were Stage 1, Zone 2, no plus disease. What does "stage" refer to in these results?
    A. Extent
    B. Location
    C. Severity

96) The most common cause of non-hereditary sensorineural hearing loss is
    A. cytomegalovirus congenital infection
    B. neurodegenerative disorder
    C. recurrent or persistent otitis media

97) A term male infant requires intubation for respiratory distress. The medications recommended for modified rapid sequence are atropine and a
    A. muscle relaxant
    B. narcotic
    C. short-acting benzodiazepine

98) An umbilical arterial catheter that is placed high (T8-T10) is more likely to be associated with complications of which system?
    A. cardiac
    B. hepatic
    C. renal

99) General principles of neonatal analgesia for invasive procedures include
    A. do not assume the infant is in pain, but assess the infant for cues of pain or stress
    B. opioid analgesia given on a scheduled basis as a preventative measure is not advised
    C. treatment with analgesics is recommended over sedation without analgesics

100) When Clindamycin is given to a neonate concomitantly with a neuromuscular blocking agent, the effect of the neuromuscular blocking agent is
    A. diminished
    B. potentiated
    C. prolonged

PRACTICE TEST ANSWER / REFERENCE

1) A nuchal translucency is done at 12 weeks that shows an increased nuchal thickening. Additional testing may include

   B. fetal echocardiogram

   REFERENCE: CHAPTER 1

2) The presence of maternal hyperglycemia places the neonate at risk for

   C. hyperinsulinemia

   REFERENCE: CHAPTER 2

3) A mother is admitted to the birthing center due to declining renal function and severe headache with visual changes. She is carrying 24 week twins and has been on bed rest for the past 8 weeks. After 48 hours the mother's headache and visual changes persist. The clinician can expect

   B. induction of labor is likely

   REFERENCE: CHAPTER 3

4) A neonate born to a mother given Demerol three hours prior to delivery is apneic and cyanotic with heart rate of 74 at one hour after birth. The initial intervention should be

   B. bag and mask ventilation

   REFERENCE: CHAPTER 4

5) What size endotracheal tube should be available to resuscitate a 36 week 2500g newborn?

   C. 3.5 mm

   REFERENCE: CHAPTER 4

6) Hydrops Fetalis involves extracellular fluid in

   A. 2 or more body compartments

   REFERENCE: CHAPTER 5

7) Following a traumatic delivery, a neonate's arm falls motionless along the side of the body and is rotated inwards. Extension of the forearm is present and grasp reflex is intact. This infant likely has

   A. Erb's Palsy

   REFERENCE: CHAPTER 6

8) To confirm or supplement obstetric dating for infants at 20-24 weeks gestation, the following should be used

   A. Ballard Newborn Maturity Rating

   REFERENCE: CHAPTER 7

9) A neonate born at 36 weeks gestation had Apgar scores of 8 and 8 and appears to be physiologically stable. The nurse notes that the infant has hiccups, frequent yawns and occasionally sneezes. These are signs of

   A. autonomic stress

   REFERENCE: CHAPTER 8

10) When following safe sleep guidelines, a baby sleeps on

    C. supine

    REFERENCE: CHAPTER 9

11) Teratogenic agents are most likely to cause birth defects when the fetus is exposed during the

    A. 4th-7th weeks of gestation

    REFERENCE: CHAPTER 10

12) What are the characteristics of a dizygotic pregnancy?

    C. 2 placentas, 2 chorions and 2 amniotic sacs

    REFERENCE: CHAPTER 11

13) The AAP recommends that opioid exposed infants remain in the hospital for a minimum of

    C. 96 hours

    REFERENCE: CHAPTER 12

14) Potential outcomes of neonates who were exposed to cocaine in utero include

    B. neurobehavior abnormalities

    REFERENCE: CHAPTER 12

15) A woman on methadone wants to breastfeed. She should be advised that

    B. she may as long as she remains in a substance abuse treatment program

    REFERENCE: CHAPTER 12

16) An 800g 26 week infant has a mean blood pressure of 20mm Hg at 12 hours of life. The most likely cause of this infant's hypotension is

    A. altered vasoreactivity

    REFERENCE: CHAPTER 13

17) When repositioning infants it is important to provide

    C. midline alignment

    REFERENCE: CHAPTER 14

18) A neutral thermal environment is the environmental temperature in which body temperature is maintained and
   A. energy expenditure is minimized
   REFERENCE: CHAPTER 15

19) Risk of blindness due to ROP in the ELBW population is
   C. > 2%
   REFERENCE: CHAPTER 16

20) After an initial resuscitation, poor perfusion continues, pulses are thready, and the neonate appears in shock. Dopamine is administered as a continuous IV infusion. The transport nurse should recognize that
   A. beneficial effects are dependent on adequate blood volume
   REFERENCE: CHAPTER 17

21) When there is a surviving multiple (twin, triplet, etc.) the team should acknowledge
   B. the difficulty this will present during the grieving process
   REFERENCE: CHAPTER 20

22) When comparing the same volume of mature human milk and premature human milk, the mature milk has less
   C. protein
   REFERENCE: CHAPTER 21

23) A two week old premature infant exhibits fussiness, gagging and poor feeding behavior. Gastroesophageal reflux (GER) is the suspected diagnosis. The nurse should know that
   C. symptoms usually respond to alterations in feeding regimen
   REFERENCE: CHAPTER 21

24) A breastfeeding mother develops redness on her right breast accompanied by fever, chills and headache. In addition to antibiotic therapy, an appropriate intervention would be
   B. continue breastfeeding to empty affected breast
   REFERENCE: CHAPTER 22

25) A breastfeeding baby should return to birth weight by how many days of life?
   B. 12-14
   REFERENCE: CHAPTER 22

26) Low urinary chloride can be caused by
   C. vomiting
   REFERENCE: CHAPTER 23

27) In the term infant the percentage of weight loss in the first 5 to 6 days is
   B. 3-5%
   REFERENCE: CHAPTER 23

28) An extremely premature neonate is hyperglycemic with a serum glucose of 250mg/dL. The provider orders a one-time does of insulin. The correct dose is
   A. 0.05 to 0.1 units/kg
   REFERENCE: CHAPTER 24

29) Calcium levels usually decline for the first 24-48 hours after birth. The nadir of neonatal calcium for a healthy term infant is
   B. 7.5 to 8.4mg/dL
   REFERENCE: CHAPTER 25

30) Regarding neonatal hypercalcemia, the upper limit of normal for serum total calcium is
   B. 11 mg/dL
   REFERENCE: CHAPTER 25

31) Which of the following is a true statement regarding neonatal hyperbilirubinemia?
   C. Newborn infants produce more bilirubin per day than adults
   REFERENCE: CHAPTER 26

32) Bronze baby syndrome is caused by phototherapy in a baby with which of the following conditions?
   A. Direct hyperbilirubinemia
   REFERENCE: CHAPTER 26

33) The primary cause of most cholestasis or conjugated hyperbilirubinemia in the NICU is
   B. prolonged exposure to parenteral nutrition
   REFERENCE: CHAPTER 26

34) The x-ray of a neonate with suspected necrotizing enterocolitis shows pneumoperitoneum. This finding is consistent with
   C. intestinal perforation
   REFERENCE: CHAPTER 27

PRACTICE TEST ANSWER / REFERENCE

35) NEC in term infants most commonly affects the
   A. colon
   REFERENCE: CHAPTER 27

36) Aminoglycosides are a factor in which renal disease category?
   A. Intrinsic
   REFERENCE: CHAPTER 28

37) Which of the following statements regarding Continuous Positive Airway Pressure (CPAP) is true?
   C. prevents alveolar and airway collapse
   REFERENCE: CHAPTER 29

38) When considering noninvasive capnography, the clinician should know that
   B. mainstream devices increase mechanical dead space
   REFERENCE: CHAPTER 30

39) Administration of supplemental oxygen is most effective in treatment for hypoxemia resulting from
   A. diffusion impairment
   REFERENCE: CHAPTER 30

40) Most apnea spells in the preterm infant are
   B. mixed
   REFERENCE: CHAPTER 31

41) Apnea of prematurity
   C. will most likely present in the first week of life
   REFERENCE: CHAPTER 31

42) Which condition increases the neonate's risk for transient tachypnea of the newborn (TTN)?
   A. Cesarean birth
   REFERENCE: CHAPTER 32

43) By 24 weeks gestation, which of the following is adequately developed to provide gas exchange in the ELBW newborn?
   A. Basic lung structure
   REFERENCE: CHAPTER 33

44) The key principle in the management of respiratory distress syndrome is to
   A. establish and maintain functional residual capacity
   REFERENCE: CHAPTER 33

45) The chest x-ray appearance of infants in early stages of bronchopulmonary dysplasia is
   A. diffuse haziness and increased density
   REFERENCE: CHAPTER 34

46) What type of mechanical ventilation appears to reduce the incidence of bronchopulmonary dysplasia and pulmonary air leak?
   C. Volume targeted ventilation
   REFERENCE: CHAPTER 34

47) When meconium aspiration syndrome is suspected, x-ray findings that would be consistent with this diagnosis are
   A. hyperinflation
   REFERENCE: CHAPTER 35

48) Approximately how many deliveries are complicated by meconium stained amniotic fluid?
   B. 10-15%
   REFERENCE: CHAPTER 35

49) The most commonly associated diagnosis with persistent pulmonary hypertension of the newborn is
   C. severe fetal hypoxemia
   REFERENCE: CHAPTER 36

50) In an effort to decrease the hemodynamic shunt in infants with persistent pulmonary hypertension of the newborn, the treatment goal is to maintain the systemic blood pressure
   B. higher than pulmonary vascular resistance
   REFERENCE: CHAPTER 36

51) The underlying pathogenesis of pulmonary hemorrhage remains unclear. Supportive treatment is recommended, including
   A. administration of packed red blood cells
   REFERENCE: CHAPTER 37

52) The precise pathophysiology underlying pulmonary hemorrhage remains uncertain. However, a predisposing condition that may initiate hemorrhage in the neonatal lung is

   B. **an alteration in the integrity of the alveolar epithelial-endothelial barrier**

   REFERENCE: CHAPTER 37

53) A chest x-ray reveals a hypertranslucent hemothorax on an asymptomatic full-term newborn 6 hours post-Caesarean delivery. The infant required positive-pressure ventilation in the delivery room. What is the appropriate management?

   A. **Close observation**

   REFERENCE: CHAPTER 38

54) At 36 hours of age a 28 week gestation premature infant is intubated and placed on a ventilator. The infant's condition gradually deteriorates with heart rate < 100bpm and blood pressure of 30/16. ABG results are pH-7.25, PaO_2-32, $PaCO_2$-58. Chest x-ray appearance is linear radiolucencies radiating from the lung helium. What is the likely diagnosis?

   C. **Pulmonary interstitial emphysema**

   REFERENCE: CHAPTER 38

55) During ECMO poor venous return to the circuit causes the pump to shut down in order to prevent

   A. **air entrapment**

   REFERENCE: CHAPTER 39

56) A full term neonate on ECMO day 5 has fluid overload. What is the expected treatment while on ECMO?

   C. **Hemofiltration**

   REFERENCE: CHAPTER 39

57) Which inotrope's effect on myocardial contractility is dependent on myocardial norepinephrine stores?

   B. **Dopamine**

   REFERENCE: CHAPTER 40

58) A newborn is diagnosed with cyanotic heart disease. Which of the following is an example of this type of congenital heart defect?

   B. **Ebstein's anomaly**

   REFERENCE: CHAPTER 41

59) What percentage of congenital heart defects are considered critical congenital heart disease requiring intervention in the first year of life?

   B. **25**

   REFERENCE: CHAPTER 41

60) 30 minutes after initiation of PGE_1 on an infant with suspected cardiac anomaly, the patient's condition worsens. Which category of lesions would the clinician be most concerned with?

   A. **Left atrial hypertension**

   REFERENCE: CHAPTER 41

61) What percentage of infants with complete atrioventricular canal have Trisomy 21?

   B. **70%**

   REFERENCE: CHAPTER 41

62) A 3500g term infant male is born to a 35 y/o G1P0 and noted to have persistent platelet counts less than 50,000. A diagnosis of neonatal alloimmune thrombocytopenia is made. Which would be an appropriate treatment for this infant?

   B. **Intravenous immunoglobulin**

   REFERENCE: CHAPTER 42

63) The occurrence of newborn hemorrhagic disease in infants who do not receive vitamin K is one out of every

   A. **200-400 infants**

   REFERENCE: CHAPTER 43

64) Which diagnostic test should be performed in all cases of suspected aortic thrombosis?

   C. **Ultrasound**

   REFERENCE: CHAPTER 44

65) A preterm infant born at 24 weeks gestation has persistent respiratory failure and pale color despite resuscitation. The initial hematocrit is 15. What test would you consider requesting to determine if fetomaternal bleeding occurred?

   C. **Kleihauer-Betke stain**

   REFERENCE: CHAPTER 45

PRACTICE TEST ANSWER / REFERENCE

66) Which condition is most associated with polycythemia?
   A. Beckwith-Weideman Syndrome
   REFERENCE: CHAPTER 46

67) The most frequent cause of thrombocytopenia in an asymptomatic neonate in the first 72 hours of life is
   C. placental insufficiency
   REFERENCE: CHAPTER 47

68) A 38-week gestation neonate is born to a HIV positive mother who has not received prenatal care. The clinician should be aware that the rate of HIV transmission from untreated infected mothers to their newborns is estimated to be between
   A. 15-40%
   REFERENCE: CHAPTER 48

69) The most common presenting symptom of early onset sepsis is
   B. respiratory distress
   REFERENCE: CHAPTER 49

70) Recent evidence reveals the drug of choice to prevent Candida infection in VLBW infants is
   B. fluconazole
   REFERENCE: CHAPTER 49

71) Congenital toxoplasmosis is most often secondary to
   A. acute maternal infection during pregnancy
   REFERENCE: CHAPTER 50

72) Which of the following descriptions describes the clinical presentation of most neonates affected by congenital syphilis?
   A. Asymptomatic
   REFERENCE: CHAPTER 51

73) If the mother of a newborn has a positive TB test and a normal chest x-ray, which of the following describes appropriate management of her infant?
   B. Do not delay discharge, but test family members for TB. Mother may breastfeed.
   REFERENCE: CHAPTER 52

74) Early case reports and case studies have documented that transplacental transmission of B. burgborferi is possible. Women who are seropositive for B. burgborferi with their first prenatal visit and at the time of delivery are more likely to have a newborn with:
   C. no adverse neonatal outcome
   REFERENCE: CHAPTER 53

75) A neonate with a moderate subarachnoid hemorrhage is being discharged. The parents are concerned about the infant's potential problems. The clinician should advise that
   C. hydrocephalus may occur
   REFERENCE: CHAPTER 54

76) According to the Volpe grading system, an intraventricular hemorrhage that occupies 10-50% of ventricular area on parasagittal view would be a
   B. Grade II
   REFERENCE: CHAPTER 54

77) Which of the following statements correctly describes seizures caused by hypoxic-ischemic encephalopathy?
   A. Seizures are often subclinical and difficult to monitor.
   REFERENCE: CHAPTER 55

78) Simultaneous fast rhythmic contractions of extremities with slower relaxation phase describes what type of neonatal seizure?
   A. Focal clonic
   REFERENCE: CHAPTER 56

79) In the neonatal brain, clinical seizures are reflective of
   A. diminished connectivity of neurons
   REFERENCE: CHAPTER 56

80) What is the most common way a developmental dislocation of the hip is diagnosed in a newborn?
   A. Physical examination
   REFERENCE: CHAPTER 58

81) An indication of congenital anomaly of the femur is
   A. a dimple on the buttocks
   REFERENCE: CHAPTER 58

82) What lab screening provides the earliest indication of osteopenia of prematurity?

   C. Serum phosphorus level

   REFERENCE: CHAPTER 59

83) Glycogen Storage Disease Type II (Pompe Disease) is associated with which of the following in the neonate?

   A. Cardiomyopathy

   REFERENCE: CHAPTER 60

84) Pyruvate dehydrogenase deficiency (PDH) is usually inherited by which pattern of inheritance?

   C. X-linked

   REFERENCE: CHAPTER 60

85) A neonate has a low T4 and elevated TSH. The appropriate next step would be

   A. begin thyroid hormone replacement therapy

   REFERENCE: CHAPTER 61

86) Small left colon syndrome can be treated with

   C. enemas

   REFERENCE: CHAPTER 62

87) Fetal and neonatal mortality is caused by stillbirths, birth asphyxia, hypoxic ischemic encephalopathy and intra-amniotic infections is most closely associated with which type of maternal diabetes?

   C. Type 2

   REFERENCE: CHAPTER 62

88) Rapid evaluation of an infant with suspected congenital adrenal hyperplasia is critical to prevent

   C. severe dehydration

   REFERENCE: CHAPTER 63

89) During a morning assessment of a 26 week gestation neonate who is now DOL #15 the clinician observes the following: distended tense abdomen, BP 30/15, poor perfusion and bloody stools. Which condition should be suspected?

   B. Necrotizing enterocolitis

   REFERENCE: CHAPTER 64

90) A term neonate who has just come off mechanical ventilation and begun enteric feedings has developed abdominal distention and bile stained emesis. An x-ray depicts distended bowel that may be granular in appearance or may show tiny bubbles. These clinical and x-ray findings are consistent with

   B. meconium ileus

   REFERENCE: CHAPTER 64

91) An infant admitted for suspected sepsis develops a red, excoriated and bleeding diaper rash, with scattered yellow pustules. In addition to keeping the area dry and clean, additional intervention should include application of

   C. barrier cream

   REFERENCE: CHAPTER 65

92) The adhesive removal method that reduces the risk of epidermal stripping in the premature infant is the use of

   C. Warm sterile water

   REFERENCE: CHAPTER 65

93) An anomaly that typically arises postnatally and demonstrates endothelial proliferation is a vascular

   C. Tumor

   REFERENCE: CHAPTER 66

94) After the initial ophthalmologic exam for a neonate in the NICU that revealed immature retina, when should the neonate be rescreened?

   B. Two weeks

   REFERENCE: CHAPTER 67

95) A 30 week gestation neonate was screened for Retinopathy of Prematurity. The findings were Stage 1, Zone 2, no plus disease. What does "stage" refer to in these results?

   C. Severity

   REFERENCE: CHAPTER 67

96) The most common cause of non-hereditary sensorineural hearing loss is

   A. cytomegalovirus congenital infection

   REFERENCE: CHAPTER 68

PRACTICE TEST ANSWER / REFERENCE

97) A term male infant requires intubation for respiratory distress. The medications recommended for modified rapid sequence are atropine and a

   A. muscle relaxant

   REFERENCE: CHAPTER 69

98) An umbilical arterial catheter that is placed high (T8-T10) is more likely to be associated with complications of which system?

   C. renal

   REFERENCE: CHAPTER 69

99) General principles of neonatal analgesia for invasive procedures include

   C. treatment with analgesics is recommended over sedation without analgesics

   REFERENCE: CHAPTER 70

100) When Clindamycin is given to a neonate concomitantly with a neuromuscular blocking agent, the effect of the neuromuscular blocking agent is

   B. potentiated

   REFERENCE: APPX A